The Book I Wish I Had Before Marriage and Divorce

The Book I Wish I Had Before Marriage and Divorce
Remodeling the Foundation That Relationships Are Built Upon

Zach Saleh

©2024 All Rights Reserved. No portion of this book may be reproduced, stored in a retrieval system, or transmitted in any form or by any means- electronic, mechanical, photocopy, recording, scanning, or other-except for brief quotations in critical reviews or articles without the prior permission of the author.

Published by Game Changer Publishing

Paperback ISBN: 978-1-963793-18-5
Hardcover ISBN: 978-1-963793-19-2
Digital: ISBN: 978-1-963793-20-8

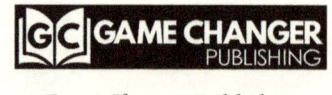

www.GameChangerPublishing.com

DEDICATION

To my kids, Zayda and Isaac, it's an honor and gift to be your father. You've been a mirror since day one reflecting back to me all the ways I can grow and be stronger. Thank you for being so generous with love and grace.

To all those I've been in a relationship with, thank you for playing a role in my life that has revealed the parts of me hidden in the shadows. I'm deeply sorry for the pain my unhealed self contributed to our experience. Please forgive me for living in brokenness and creating more pain. Thank you for playing the role that you did.

To my family and closest friends who are doing life beside me, walking beside each one of you is a precious gift. I am humbled by the presence and life you bring to my soul.

Brett, you led me through the wrestle of my ego and into the I AM.

Tyler, Tim and Brandon, thank you for being my brothers from another mother.

To everyone who has ever caused me pain, thank you for being my teachers.

– Zachary Saleh

Read This First

Just to say thanks for buying and reading my book, I would like to give you a free bonus gift, no strings attached!

Get Ready to Change Your Life, Scan Now:

The Book I Wish I Had Before Marriage and Divorce

Remodeling the Foundation That Relationships Are Built Upon

Zach Saleh

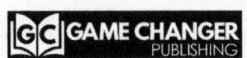

www.GameChangerPublishing.com

To The Younger Me

Dear Zachary,

You've been through a lot. First, push pause and acknowledge it's not been all rainbows and butterflies as you're skilled at minimizing the effects the last decade have had on you. The amount of pain you've experienced—you probably aren't even aware of quite yet. It's going to show its face through triggers, insecurities, and unspoken vendettas. Everything you've encountered, believe it or not, you've helped create. You'd be surprised to hear that your hands have fashioned this life. Now, I'm not saying it's all your fault, but kinda. Your unconscious patterns on autopilot have attracted and made this whole mess you call life. It's *your* life, so at any moment you choose, you can flip the script and write a killer plot twist when you're ready to reveal and heal the hurt little boy driving this ship. Unpack all baggage from your relationships and what you carried into them. Really tough, but well worth it and fruitful if you're intentional about it. Heal the pain points and the narratives they carry in your heart first. Then, get clear on these four ideas, and your relationships will never be the same in romance, friendship, and even business.

Moving forward, healthy chemistry (not based on toxic behavior) is good to want. You're a connecting human, so don't apologize for that, but also get clear on good, healthy chemistry, my guy. Values aren't a catchphrase, nor are they taught clearly, so I'm gonna teach you how to find yours and how the hell to live by them. There is a little boy captaining your ship and he needs your help navigating life. Your inner values being lived by are the compass and rudder he so desperately needs to get where he's going. Learn the art of walking well through conflict, both inner and outside of yourself. And yes, it's a cultivated skill worthy of your efforts. I'll give you some formulas and lenses to see clearly how to manage conflict.

Lastly, it may seem trivial, but trust me: set and manage crystal clear expectations for yourself and others. Don't apologize to anyone if others can't hang with getting clear on expectations. Boundaries will be formed, which will create tons of safety, and I know deep down that we all need that. Unapologetically, focus on these four points like a stickler, unwavering in any form. They will change your life if they are adopted as the pillars of all connections. I'm proud of you. You should be proud of yourself right now, even in this season. Ignore this wisdom if you wanna go back to a mystery relationship lifestyle, or lean in and treat this as an intentional life-changing experience… because it will be if you apply this gold. Make your pain worth it.

Table of Contents

Introduction 1

Section 1 – The Blind Spot 5
    Chapter 1 – Dating is Dumb and Why Most Marriages Fail 7
    Chapter 2 – You Are the Problem (+ the Solution) 15

Section 2 – Playing For Keeps 31
    Chapter 3 – Values: What Are They and How Do They Change Everything? 33
    Chapter 4 – Conflict Management: Fighting With Soft Gloves 47
    Chapter 5 – Chemistry: Ya Feel Me? (Insert Side Eye) 69
    Chapter 6 – Expectations: Bids, Booty Calls and Boundaries (#expectations) 79

Section 3 – Exit 97
    Chapter 7 – What if I'm Done? 99
    Chapter 8 – Wisdom From Painful Endings 123
    Chapter 9 – Prove This Wrong 137

Introduction

It's not so much about your relationship status as it is about the lens through which you look at relationships. Honestly, if people read and applied these truths before getting married, I'm sure divorce rates would plummet by at least 30-40%. However, that's not why I wrote this book—it wasn't to save marriages. **Years ago, I made a vow to myself that I'd write this book as if I were reading it before I got married... and divorced.** Perhaps not to shield myself and others from the pain of regret, but to provide a shortcut for others to what took me 18 years to learn. This book is all substance; there are no side dishes like green beans or mashed potatoes. Can you imagine being able to go back in time and hand yourself a book? "Zach, stay away from these people," or "Don't betray yourself in this way," or "Heal this pain before you think about pursuing that person." I created this for myself as a gift for all the pain my heart has endured. I write this for the Zachary I was back then because he didn't know what he didn't know.

If you're tired of the same old relational experiences, open your mind to a new perspective that looks beyond the surface-level insights given around relationships. This is for those tired of snorkeling in the shallow end of superficial dating/marriage advice. There's a lot of gold in this book that has been intentionally harvested during my reach for the DNA of legitimate, sustainable relationships. People have different opinions on what makes great paintings historically notable. That's because art is subjective. Truth, however, ages like fine wine or delectable cheese.

I've made plenty of messes in my own life and in the lives of others, relationally speaking. Consider this the confession of someone who's been on both sides of the curtain of marriage and divorce—and everything in between. **The intention of this book is to help you redefine the inventory that will either make or break a relationship.** I will be the first to admit I wouldn't wish divorce on anyone, but I also believe there's a time and a place when even a good relationship might need to end based on its lack of key ingredients. I also know that some people end their relationships too quickly, often merely because they were ill-equipped, even though it could have been successful. So, whether you're trying to decide if you should stay or go, I invite you on a journey of intentionality.

Consider this: who you are becoming is more important than the status of your relationship.

One Midwest morning, as I was driving behind a fellow on the highway in the left lane, I smirked, realizing he had no clue his left blinker was on— he had clearly forgotten. Something inside whispered, *Look down.* To my humble surprise, I saw my own left blinker blinking, my hypocrisy staring back. The irony was that we both made the same mistake, but my arrogant arse was the only one judging. So, with the ironic stick in my own eye judging the splinter in others, I offer a posture. At the end of each chapter, there is a question or opportunity to look into your own life and examine how you might have your own blinker on.

Get curious about your story regarding past relationship experiences. Push pause on the narrative you've always internally maintained about your partner, your pain, and yourself. Imagine yourself in a courtroom where you're accustomed to adopting the self-directed posture of a prosecuting attorney. Perhaps instead, take on the objective viewpoint of a juror characterized by curiosity rather than repetitive conclusions. **Curiosity is your new posture, and this lens will change many of the conclusive beliefs in your purview.**

SECTION 1
THE BLIND SPOT

"It's admirable and kinda sad we keep creating painful endings, yet never change the lenses through which we perceive relationships." - ZJS

CHAPTER ONE

Dating is Dumb and Why Most Marriages Fail

That's right! It seems like everything we're doing isn't working. There's a 60% chance your marriage will eventually fail, so why would you do that to yourself? That's easy—we're foolish, and we desperately want our connections to work. But what if I told you that the chance of success could be 80-90% if we flip the script? We're the ones putting these ingredients into the bowl and blaming the outcome, not the recipe. It makes no sense.

Have you ever traveled internationally? If you have, you'll go to plug in your charger overseas and realize it doesn't fit the outlet. In fact, you'll find you need an adapter to make a connection. We are wired for connection, so seeking connection with other humans is literally by design. The problem is that we're going about trying to plug into connection in an unsustainable way, which only results in shocking pain (pun intended). There might be some dad jokes here, so if it's too much for your circuits or if you get your wires crossed, let's connect offline.

Before a major truth is introduced to your belief system, one must reveal the lie it is meant to replace. Everything society, culture, and even your family have taught you about qualifying a relationship is somewhat wrong. I'm dead ass serious. It's off by a nautical mile, which is longer than a normal mile for some reason.

Becky was raised Catholic and always attended mass. "A class act" was a keen description of her character. Tyler's brawn and wit kept him at the top of the proverbial food chain, and every girl was smitten. His responsible attitude as a young man kept him above reproach in most things in life. On paper, one would hesitantly admit that they seemed like the perfect match aesthetically. Their shared desire for a house on Nantucket and four beautiful children was ideal and attainable. After three years of dating, he popped the question, and they were on their way.

Full stop. This is garbage, and we all know it. But for whatever emotionally based reasons, we place ourselves in these stories. It's like a painting that's two strokes away from a dumpster fire, and I haven't even begun to squeeze the lime for citrus.

The reality is that the logical, straightforward answer is sometimes the worst possible solution. Picture two parents from an Eastern culture picking out their teenager's future spouse, riddled with required qualifications. They do their best, only to find the teen can't reconcile the two different lenses: their own parents' perception of the prospects versus their own. The logic without fail comes forth: "He's a doctor from a good family who has a good reputation. He is motivated, quite respectful, and will bring honor to our family." All checks out, right? It's an exaggeration to compare American dating or marriage to how Eastern-cultured families pick out a suitable spouse, but in reality, it's actually damn close.

The answer won't make sense unless you realize how deeply ingrained the deception is in our brains. We were mostly taught these by our family, friends, and cultural opinions, all being broadcast around us in perfect unison.

I want you to look at your previous relationships like a movie, and your job is to sit back and provide commentary on what was going through your mind at the time. It's going to be hilarious, super obnoxious, and maybe even emotional. The key is to pop some popcorn, pour a drink of your choice, and leave self-criticism and accusations of any type at the door. Push play, and let's do the damn thing because I'm right here, and this is so freaking worth the ROI (return on investment). YW (you're welcome).

You're quite possibly going to attract the relationship you've always wanted after reading and applying the lenses provided in this book. But first, we have to get you to unlearn some outlooks that are creating painful outcomes. I won't waste any time trying to put these in a specific order because, honestly, it won't matter.

> *"You're quite possibly going to attract the relationship you've always wanted after reading and applying the lenses provided in this book. But first, we have to get you to unlearn some outlooks that are creating painful outcomes."*

It doesn't take more than a few minutes of swiping on dating apps or interviewing random people out on the town to see some common denominators of what people are basing their "match criteria" on. Here are a few to reveal the landscape of our current relationship culture (cue satirical grin).

Some dating profile statements commonly found:

- Don't talk to me unless you're 6 ft. tall. I want to make D1 babies.
- Take me to all the sports games; I love sports.
- I want a swole mate.
- I'm spiritual but not religious, and I love to travel.
- My personality type is ENFJ, and I'm fluent in sarcasm.
- I enjoy cooking, music, and almost anything outdoors.
- Must spend time with family and friends.
- Hopeless romantic who enjoys simple things.
- I believe in tolerance and equality.
- Small business owner, songwriter, and side hustler.
- Looking for someone self-aware, with integrity and kindness.
- Amuse me; preferably, don't live with your parents.
- Looking for someone to build a family with and go on adventures too.
- Do you want to talk about food science, punk rock, or film?
- Never been married/no kids, so let's travel.
- I like dogs, baseball, and people with a sense of humor.
- I'm a full-time parent, and my kids will always come first.

You might say, "Zach, I don't do the apps, so this doesn't apply to me." Listen, Carl, this is a snapshot into our reality, and you're not above the rest of the class. Unfortunately, these are the criteria people are basing their pursuit of connection on, even if they're committed to it. They are all built to fail from the start, as they're based on three things.

Commonalities, Circumstances and Toxic Chemistry

We create a little chemistry by revealing some of our personality traits, such as being funny, sarcastic, or witty. We add some spice by sharing activities we like—travel, yoga, or cooking, to appeal to their senses. Then, we describe our current and future circumstances that we are experiencing or wish to experience one day. This encapsulates all three lenses through which we look for connection. "OMG, you're a foodie? I love good food." "You're Jewish, Muslim, or Christian? My parents will love you." "You're attractive, so let's pursue a relationship and see where this goes." It's going to the same place the Titanic currently rests.

Look at your last relationship or two. Didn't you base the pursuit of connection on one or all three of these "Cs" (**Commonalities, Circumstances** and Toxic **Chemistry**)? What if I told you these are the wrong lenses, but we still use them, like sitting at a stoplight with black and white lenses over our eyes? You can bet dollars to donuts that there will be accidents and unnecessary traffic jams (pain and patterns).

Most of these relationships end up being transactional and unsustainable. Harsh, maybe? If you're here for fluff, try cotton candy. If you want real, it's as authentic as my mom's hummus. My daughter might even be willing to sell you the recipe. #capitalism #youngentrepreneurs

Today's approach to relationships often starts with good intentions, but it's the equivalent of putting water in your gas tank. As soon as it starts, it's going to ruin the engine and it's not going anywhere. (Please don't do this; it's not a challenge, and yes, I have to clarify so that someone doesn't sue me.) Maybe a better example would be people who pull their Tesla up to a gas pump. It's worth a watch; you'll feel smarter.

Can you imagine what your life would be like if relationships, marriage, or even friendships were no longer based on these three things?

We look for **Commonalities,** such as similar beliefs or outlooks on specific topics like politics, morals, or religious ideologies. Some might say politics on several sides have become their own religion nowadays. A partner who safely challenges our perspectives will likely cause healthy growth—if you're into that kind of thing. It's all about how they go about it. Commonalities, such as hobbies or frequent activities, are often given more value relationally than they should be. You might love working out, walking your dog, or playing pickleball, but you can always invite someone into those activities later. Basing attraction or the willingness to pursue a connection on having the same taste in music or similar lifestyles is madness. It's like holding a lit birthday candle in the middle of a storm and wondering why it was snuffed out. These hobbies or interests shift over time, and there's no reason to base a connection on them unless you want to lessen your chances of success.

Symptomatic **Circumstances** you might prefer: their financial success, educational background, or things they own, etc., play a role. He's an engineer at the top firm on the East Coast, she's a successful nurse at a well-known hospital, he's a pro athlete—you get the drift. These can be pleasurable attributes to have or maybe a distinct preference, but we often let them dictate the pursuit right out of the gate. Life can literally change in an instant, and when we base our relationship pursuit on circumstances that can shift with the wind, it's dangerous at best. When that circumstance shifts, as all eventually do, what then becomes of the relationship?

> *"Life can literally change in an instant, and when we base our relationship pursuit on circumstances that can shift with the wind, it's dangerous at best."*

Chemistry is a necessity, but when it's based on push-pull toxic wounded behaviors, it actually perpetuates pain. For some reason, people complain about daddy issues or mommy wounds in the opposite sex, yet they perpetuate their own pain by not addressing those parental wounds that have profoundly shaped the shit out of their identity. Single women, hyper-INDEPENDENT, doing everything in a relationship and forgetting themselves and their well-being in the process, attract hyper-DEPENDENT men who want their partner to mother them while being passive and entitled. Consider the man who could do no wrong as a child and gives only breadcrumbs in his interactions, while she chases him down only to affirm her childhood neglect. Unhealthy, unbalanced masculine/feminine dynamics attract opposites. Attraction is absolutely necessary, but it has to be coupled with healthy behaviors that reveal good character and loving actions. Looking back at previous connections with curiosity, ask yourself what the chemistry was based on and whether it was healthy.

Looking at your current connection or last relationship(s), did you not base the pursuit of connection on one, if not all, three of these "Cs"?

What if I told you **these are the wrong questions,** but we still internally ask them:

- *What do we have in Common?*

- *Do I like and desire their Circumstance? (Meaning where you are currently in life and where you are both individually going?)*
- *Do we have Chemistry?*

This is revealing your version of the three "Cs." Look for how they apply to your current pursuit of what you look for in a partner.

CHAPTER TWO

You Are the Problem (+ the Solution)

No matter if you're single, married, or going through a divorce, remember this. Your current or previous partner is here to reveal to you the unhealed parts of you that are out of alignment. Any pain that you are experiencing with this partner can be a gift if you posture your heart right and process what this pain is actually trying to show you. Now, I'm no fan of self-deprecation or choosing to be a doormat. But this is a real, heart-filled invitation to look at what is causing or has caused you pain and process it well. You might say, "Zachary, it's clearly their fault," or "They're easily causing the issues in the relationship." Well, if you're willing to hear a hard truth, here's one about me.

> *"Any pain that you are experiencing with this partner can be a gift if you posture your heart right and process what this pain is actually trying to show you."*

I won't tell you that I was married after meeting someone 110 days later because I threw out all logic and thought I was doing the right thing.

I won't disclose that we never even dated, and I was so hungry to be a husband to someone and do life with them that I ignored every passing piece of advice given to me to simply push pause. Every red flag was present that could be, and yet, with forward motion, I ran deeper into the relationship. I would be lying if I didn't say things went wrong immediately, and I doubled down for fear of shame—shame of being wrong and shame of leaving her like everyone else had.

It would take two years before I actually considered leaving the relationship. Wouldn't you know she got pregnant? Well, I'm not going anywhere, as I made vows while growing up I'd never get divorced or have my kids go through a divorce. It's time to make it work. We stayed married for eight years. This book isn't about how I escaped the Alcatraz of relationships, or how my ex is such a terrible person, or the typical accusations like they're a narcissist. **It's quite the opposite. (I was the problem, + the solution.)**

I created, to an extent, most of my own pain. My unhealed wounds or emotional traumas built a sail that would passively guide me straight into a harbor of pain. Until I was willing to listen, the pain would repeat itself over and over, not only in that relationship, but in most relationships after it. Those childhood pains created beliefs in my heart that never showed their faces but led me to recreate my subconscious beliefs in reality. I realized that until I actually healed, this wouldn't stop being my experience. Our subconscious must, in fact, attract or recreate these scenarios as our brains desperately love one thing in the name of creating safety—repetition.

During the last two years of marriage, I went into every facet of healing I could get my hands on, from counseling, therapy, and men's retreats to life coaching and everything in between. I was all in. I became an inner healing growth mindset junky. I spent more time and money than most do on their Master's degrees. After two and a half years of this inner healing pursuit, I was finally willing to lose everything, including my friends, my family support, or even my own life, rather than let things stay the same. So finally, I ended the relationship. I wished to God someone would have warned me, *Hey, just because you're ending the relationship, you're not alone, and you're not a bad person. Zach, you're still worthy of love. There's grace to be found here.* Here's a map that'll help you navigate the mountain you are about to climb.

If you've decided to leave your current relationship or to stay in it, that's your prerogative. I have no judgments either way if you fix it or not. What I will tell you is that both are equally hard in their own ways. So choose your hard. Either way, if you dig into the aha moments that will surface as you read this book, your life will never look the same.

My previous partner and I were standing in the kitchen having an argument, and our voices were raised. After a pause in the argument, my kids came running down the hallway, screaming, "Daddy, Daddy, please stop. Mom, please stop arguing. Dad, please stop." And I realized at that moment, in the most sobering of realizations, my children were living my childhood to a degree. We were both responsible in our own ways for co-creating the life we had in that moment.

Fast forward from that time on, we would experience two separations. And after the second, the relationship would finally end. A few years into the relationship, I realized my heart was breaking. I kept renegotiating contracts with my own heart. If she does this, then we'll separate, or if she does that or says this, then I'll end the relationship. If she crosses this boundary, then that's it; *I'm gone, pecan*. What I was really doing was moving the threshold further and further down the line.

This was all in the name of self-preservation, yet ironically, it created self-betrayal. I made a vow as a young man, having been raised in a volatile household where emotions would change like temperatures in the Midwest. I said I'd never get a divorce, no matter what. I'll do it right, and I'll raise my kids in a peaceful home. Little did I know that inner vow would hold me in shame, obligation, and in paralyzing fear for almost a decade. I was petrified that one day, another man would hold my kids on his lap. But God forbid that my son and daughter would call another man "Father," or that my kids would resent me for the rest of their lives.

> *"Little did I know that inner vow would hold me in shame, obligation, and in paralyzing fear for almost a decade."*

It's amazing how we can justify the pain that we're in for fear of experiencing even worse pain. In reality, every relationship in your life is there to act as a mirror. It's there to literally reveal how you truly perceive yourself. We train people how to treat us. Ironically, it's up to us to love ourselves well and put up a boundary if we don't like what we're experiencing.

When I was younger, without realizing this until I was in my 30s, I used humor as an escape in the midst of fear. I would make a joke because I wanted everyone to be happy or because I could feel conflict arising, or it was an easy emotional out. So, out of a survival mechanism that I created to feel safe, the jokester was created. My personality was formed out of my personal reality. Little did I know that little traits I would identify with would end up becoming a crutch and a mechanism that I would have to part ways if I didn't want to continue experiencing pain. Beliefs were formed as a young child that would one day actually form blind spots. These blind spots in our personalities are easy to see from an outside perspective, especially if you're someone else. But I didn't know what I didn't know, and I had no clue I didn't know it.

Believe it or not, you're the same. You see, in order to get to know your blind spots, you must first reverse-engineer your triggers. **Your triggers reveal the pain that you're afraid of experiencing because that pain you used to experience has a meaning to it that you assigned.** We know that science has proven that it's not the event that just causes the pain. It's the meaning that we assign to moments about ourselves. We assign meanings to every single event in our life. It will surprise you if you ask yourself what you conclude internally after each conflict or experience in a relationship. **And that meaning created a belief. And that belief creates a future blind spot that then creates, believe it or not, pain once again.**

> *"It's the meaning we conclude about ourselves in the moment of pain."*

Part of this book is to invite you into making unconscious parts of you conscious, bringing the autopilot to the surface and grabbing the wheel while **realizing,** *Oh, I keep experiencing this pain because of these belief patterns.* It's one thing to heal the pain that we've experienced in our lives, but it's another to actually absorb the belief system that creates that pain over and over in our lives. It would eventually take three massive heartbreaks for me to finally push pause enough to truly examine not only the childhood wounds that kept creating that pain for myself but how that belief system was showing up today. **Healing is a beautiful thing, and it will be experienced to the level we are intentional about cultivating space for it to happen.**

It's not by accident that you are reading this. You're here to do work. So ask yourself this: **What are things I want to see change in my current or future romantic relationship?**

There's no physical way that you can read this book while contemplating with brutal honesty and remain in the same state that you were in before. You will bring forth answers that have been sitting dormant inside you for years. They may reveal many sobering truths about yourself, and that's ok. You will then become responsible to your heart for enacting those insights that came to light. **The action of stewarding self-realization is what actual self-love is supposed to look like.**

LOOK AT HOW POWERFUL YOU ARE!

If you can make a mess, you can create a masterpiece. Look at the last 5 to 10 years of your life and ask yourself, what are some of the messes that I've made, small and big? Look at the biggest mistakes you've ever made in your life and chew on the fact that you helped create not only this giant mess, but it reveals how powerful you actually are. If you can be willing, celebrate that reality. So in turn, if you were to make the unconscious conscious, you could create a powerful masterpiece just as easily as you could create those messes. It's hard to imagine, but everywhere you go, there you are. If you get anything out of this book, this chapter is all I genuinely care about at the end of the day. It's that you are not what happened to you, but what you consciously create. This is a lens worth putting up to your eyes, and looking at every aspect of your life, especially in connection with other people, you are helping create every experience you have. If you don't like the experience, you don't have to experience it again.

> *"Look at the biggest mistakes you've ever made in your life and chew on the fact that you helped create not only this giant mess, but it reveals how powerful you actually are."*

You don't have to repeat it. You can put up a boundary; that's up to you. If You do like the experience, You get to double down on that and go, Wow, how did I help create this beautiful, fulfilling thing? One of my favorite places to have moments of clarity or "aha" moments, if you will, is the shower. You get in, there's no phone, there's nothing to distract you, and it's just you in the water right on your head.

One day, I asked myself, *Zach, what's the healthiest relationship you've ever had?* And I realized at that moment that I had never actually experienced a fulfilling, safe, and healthy relationship. To say it was sobering was an understatement. In fact, it was downright embarrassing and shameful. Immediately, I looked in the mirror in my heart, and I thought, *Wow, how did you get here, Zachary?* And that night, I began to reverse-engineer every relational experience I had ever had. I was the common denominator in every single one of them. What's funny is even though I looked at how badly I was treated or how unhealthy my partner showed up in each toxic cycle. Regardless, I was the constant. Messes had been made in my life, and I saw my contribution in every single one for what it was.

I acknowledged my power in the creation of my messes.

I was the one across from them on the merry-go-round, spinning it just as powerfully as they were because I was involved. That was my contribution. This revelation would then propel me into what caused me to show up the way I did in relationships with brutal honesty. I was legitimately committed to rescuing others and being abandoned emotionally. I had no idea, but I was running to the victim card. I would posture myself as a rescuer who would only experience pain. At the cost of me, they would experience love. Because in my mind, if I would love them enough, then I would be worthy of love. **P.S. That model of love is not sustainable.** That moment you realize you're committed to being a victim or rescuer is a sobering one. **(Yes, whatever you're experiencing is what you're committed to.) The truth will set you free, but first, it will piss you off.**

There's an idea called the drama triangle. It's presented in a book called Escaping the Victim Trap. And as I read it, I would look at everyone around me in my life and go, Oh, my gosh, they totally do this or they do that. I can't believe I've never seen this before. And then I placed the whole thing as a giant mirror in front of me and went, How the hell am I the one who does this? (With the intention of proving it true.)

Back to three-sided shapes (triangles) and their relevance to *you*. There's the **victim**, the **rescuer**, and the **prosecutor**. I lived most of my life as a rescuer and a victim without having any clue. And in the midst of any conflict, I would immediately try to rescue or, without realizing it, run to the victim card and victimize myself or place myself in the posture of receiving abusive or neglectful responses. Then, when I feared that was about to happen, I'd go to the prosecutor so I could avoid the pain altogether.

It's freaking hilarious today in pop psychology that everyone's ex is a narcissist, but no one wants to talk about their contribution to that cycle. No one wants to take ownership of how they allow, permit, and help create toxic dynamics. The first time someone shows you who they are, believe them and act accordingly. You might have had painful events take place in your life physically, emotionally, and spiritually, but those do not define who you are as a person. You may have been victimized, but that does not mean you are a victim, especially at your core identity. You can acknowledge the impact of others' actions and still take ownership of your contribution. It doesn't have to be one or the other.

> *"You might have had painful events take place in your life physically, emotionally, and spiritually, but those do not define who you are as a person."*

When we allow our pain to define our identity, it's almost as if we become emotional hypochondriacs. We assign the meaning of our painful event and we put an anchor right there and we say, "I'm not moving. This is who I am. Look what you did to me." We are immediately in that moment, **surrendering all of our power**. I hate that, for others, the injustice of feeling powerless. They deserve better, you deserve more.

My invitation to you is to take back your power by owning and identifying your contribution to your painful experience in some way, shape or form. When you do that, you raise the anchor to your ship out of feeling stuck, and you open up the sail toward actual healing, finally departing from the identity of victimhood. This is by far the most important lens shift of your life. Are you tired of life happening *to* you, not *for* you?

Applying the lens of all things ownership over my life story has been the most empowering and sobering gift I've ever received. My life mission is to invite others to embody the lens of extreme personal ownership and radical honesty. If you're experiencing pain, it can be leveraged into fertilizer. Don't waste it. I love this work, and I can't wait to hear your story of personal growth.

If you don't like it, it's legitimately up to you to change it.

Reflection Questions:

1. **What model of love were you indirectly taught by your guardians or parents?**

   _____

   _____

   _____

   _____

   _____

2. **Whose love did you crave and never get? And what did you have to become to get it?**

3. **How does this same model show up in your relationships, or do you overcompensate?**

4. What's your idea of a solid, safe, and fulfilling relationship?

5. What does that relationship actually look like?

6. How would you have to show up differently to intentionally cultivate the type of relationship you desire?

_____
_____
_____
_____
_____
_____

7. Why do you think these things in a relationship are important to you?

_____
_____
_____
_____
_____
_____

8. On a scale of 1 to 10, if you desire a partner who is an 8, 9, or 10 in terms of value, what kind of person would you need to become to attract or secure that partner?

_____

_____

_____

_____

_____

(SIDE NOTE: Some people aim for a 6 or 7. They settle for a 5 and put the car in cruise control, only to be served with divorce papers 10-15 years later.)

9. How do you operate in each role of the drama triangle?

_____

_____

_____

_____

_____

10. Are you willing to be proactive when drama ensues and own how you're showing up with sincerity and actually changing?

_____
_____
_____
_____
_____
_____

11. How am I recreating my childhood in my current and previous relationships?

_____
_____
_____
_____
_____
_____

SECTION 2
PLAYING FOR KEEPS

"It's four concepts, four pillars upon which to build a fulfilling relationship. It has been said, 'A fool builds his house on sand, and a wise man builds upon the rock.' I would call these ideas a solid foundation, worthy of being built upon." -ZJS'

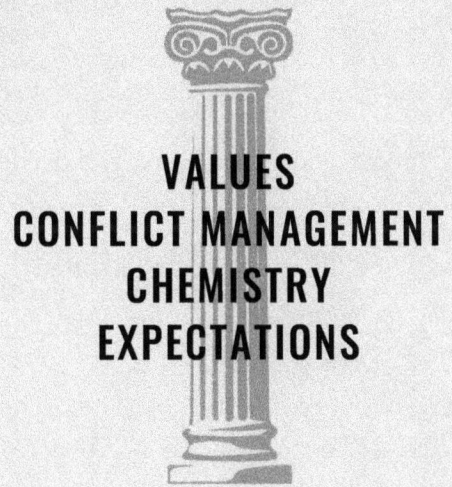

**VALUES
CONFLICT MANAGEMENT
CHEMISTRY
EXPECTATIONS**

CHAPTER THREE

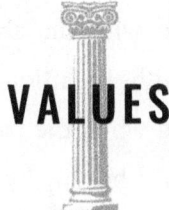

VALUES

What Are They and How Do They Change Everything?

My parents were barely making ends meet financially, and going out to eat was quite the treat. We were at a Chinese buffet (Dad's favorite), and I remember seeing my dad secretly sneak over to the waitress and discretely point at the family next to us. He was quietly covering their check. I didn't know why, but somehow I knew what he was doing, and it pierced my soul. I witnessed generosity in secret, and it created a moment I'll never forget. There was no acknowledgment by anyone and no selfie video about the act. I remember thinking no one saw it or knew what happened but me. At that moment, no trophy or award could paint my dad in a better light. I could hear my inner voice say, *Be a generous man, be like Dad.*

To say I value generosity at my core is an accurate statement. There's an energetic high, a fulfillment, and even a selfish payoff that one gets from being generous. Maybe it's partially a committed desire to never feel financially powerless again and, on the flip side, to bless others in the process. It's like a positive form of control, maybe.

Sometimes, a value is a characteristic that's near and dear to your heart, produced by layers of meanings.

What are values? Values are like the rudder and compass of a well-built ship. Both are designed with the ability to steer and direct one towards one's destination with intentionality. The direction of your connections will be redirected when the pain of conflict and heartbreak takes place. You may get tossed heavily by the storms and waves of life, but by operating on your values, you ultimately find yourself back on course. I would submit that most of us are walking around not truly clear on what our values are. Sometimes, in order to efficiently define something as important as values, **it's easier to describe what they're not for clarity's sake.**

Values are not to be mistaken with **morals, commonalities, roles, or entities**. For example, one might say they value their marriage, their family, or their religion/faith. Those would be **considered entities**, not values. I'm not negating things you might care about, but I genuinely want to help you define values and how those values show up in your life.

It's important for a few reasons to get clear on one's values, even in the conscious community, as I see people mistake spirituality for values and wonder why their relationships aren't clear. Oh, he loves to meditate and work out. He's adventurous, and we walk our dogs together. OMG, Becky! No, those are **commonalities**. And those can shift with time or even the breeze. They are a death threat to a relationship. If you base any decision on such ideas as commonalities, they're convenient and feel-good aspects of a relationship, nothing more. The icing on the cake, so to speak. "Hey, do you like hummus? Oh, snap. I love hummus. Get in, my little baba ganoush; we're going shopping!"

> *"If you base any decision on such ideas as commonalities, they're convenient and feel-good aspects of a relationship, nothing more."*

Some say they want to be around people who are good and living a "decent, honest life." Morality is fine, but **values are somewhat of a hill you're willing to die on, characteristically speaking.** They are the adjectives that describe a human experience, a characteristic embodied, and an action that brings fulfillment and safety to you. You might be a completely different human in every aspect of life, but if you value personal ownership and authenticity, you and I would share those two values.

You are someone's son or daughter. **That is a role.** Maybe you're a parent, sibling, or friend. You might have a job that you've mistakenly centered your identity around, like an athlete, one injury away from a life crisis. Those are **roles**. They're an expression of who you are, a hat you might wear.

"Who are you?" When asked this question, we typically respond with what we do—our roles. It's easy as a human to mask our identity in our roles. In fact, I'd argue that finding our relevance or value as a person in the societal roles we play is the easiest thing. This can be seen in jobs like that of an engineer who designs important structures, a nurse who saves lives daily, or an entrepreneur who employs hundreds of people. This is such a double whammy because, on the one hand, it can be absolutely fulfilling to show up in our roles. The problem presents itself when we have a hard time defining who we are outside of these affirming roles.

They're opportunities and places to show the rest of us the expression of who you are.

I digress from the roles, but now you understand they're not at all values. **When your roles shift in a few decades, it will have a radical effect on your identity, but values will only grow, stack, and develop with time.** It will serve you to base who you are around your core values and how they show up in life vs. your roles when empty nest syndrome happens or you are no longer in that professional position.

Our voids create our values. Take a moment to pause while writing down in list format your friends and romantic relationships that have caused you pain in the last ten years. Looking past the surface, what characteristics caused you pain? What are some common denominators or recurring themes worth weighing out? I thought I knew what my values were until sitting across from my life coach during a coaching session. He's in the midst of sharing a personal story when, all of a sudden, I begin reflecting on the relationship I had just left, and it hits me like a left hook to the jaw. I said, "Excuse me, one second." I grabbed my journal and wrote out the following statement: *"I value communication and extreme ownership."* To describe HOW both of these "showed up" or define the expression of said values, I wrote:

1. *Communication*: shows up with honesty and authentic vulnerability.

2. *Extreme ownership*: shows up like a willingness to take ownership with proactive growth. (It's important to note how a value shows up in life, as your value for loyalty might overlap or show up in the way my value for honesty does.)

These voids or painful dynamics created these two values written above. Two things that caused me the most pain while in relationships. My previous partners, on the other side of the relationship, lacked clear, authentic, safe, and honest communication. Also, there was the pain of dealing with a lack of ownership that would result in proactive, self-motivated growth. During conflict, one partner would completely shut down and verbally appease, while the next relationship would become extremely aggressive, unapproachable, and defensive. The pain of desiring clear, safe communication and not receiving it has instilled in me a deep value for experiencing such communication in a relationship. These voids created my value for communication that showed up with authenticity.

When I asked a partner to look at something that was affecting our relationship, they either appeased me with empty assurances or victimized excuses why they couldn't look in the mirror. There wasn't growth sought after or **ownership** of any kind when invited to look in the mirror, especially not proactively. It may sound harsh or oversimplifying, but my relationships were revealing what was painfully being ignored inside me. **What pain was being ignored kept the rudder and compass of my relational ship unused and out of sync. That's on me.**

The painful events that you have experienced over and over, when processed and healed, **reveal your values in the voids they leave behind**. If you have not healed or processed those painful events, they are still merely triggers, and they will control your emotions and dictate your experience. If this were put into a spectrum, then negative would be on the left of ZERO, which is pain and trauma, and the healed processed version would be to the right of ZERO. When pain is remedied, and insight is gained into the wound and the healthy receipt of the opposite, that is a value.

Our pain, if healed and processed properly, will give us insight into what we value and **want to experience in connection.** In fact, it will be uniquely fulfilling when two people with shared values experience connection in life. This can be in friendship and in romantic relationships. Now, I'm not saying you can't have a good relationship with anyone if you don't have shared values. In fact, you can have such a thing. It would be great if at least you understood and honored one another's values. It would be better if you had an overlapping value or three.

> *"In fact, it will be uniquely fulfilling when two people with shared values experience connection in life."*

We need to know what value looks like for someone and how it actually shows up in life. That'll give some real applicable clarity. You could value consideration, and it shows up in a specific way. I can have the same value of being considerate, but it completely manifests in a way you never thought of. Thus, the meaning of that value is different for both of us, but we share it. The opposite may manifest where we don't share the same values, but you value integrity, and I value dependability, but they show up the same. Often, circumstances showcase one reason for a relationship ending when, in fact, it's dissected; a lack of shared values is truly the reason it broke. (Mismanaged expectations and unshared values are the top two reasons most connections end).

Take your pain points you listed a moment ago. Now ask, *What's the exact opposite of my painful experience?* **The healthy opposite of what caused you pain is potentially a core value.** Everyone has a different way of coming to a conclusion regarding values, but at the end of the day, your voids and your pain create your values. Being aligned with a friend or life partner in shared values can lead to significant traction and breakthroughs in any area of life. Be careful; we're talking about power couple status here.

Sitting across from a married couple who shared the same value of loyalty, it became clear that the same value manifested completely differently for each of them. For her, loyalty manifests in one way. For the husband, it wasn't the same at all. They both valued loyalty and that much was clear. However, some of their lenses were different and needed clarification on how they showed up for one another. It was downright healing for them both to clarify how loyalty shows up in relationships and what that looks like for them as individuals. Tears were shed, and understanding on both sides brought forth a deeper emotional connection.

> *"It's just as important to identify how your values show up in relationships as it is to know what you actually value."*

A few other helpful formulas for getting clear on your values are as follows: Ask yourself, if you were able to, what **red flags or unspoken rules** you have when it comes to friendships or relationships. These characteristics reveal what is truly meaningful to you. Is it that you need communication if someone is going to be late for our hangout? Or is it that lying is a complete deal-breaker? Ask yourself: *What are the unspoken rules that are deal-breakers in a relationship? Which characteristic creates that experience?* Clarify these points.

For some, it may be honesty. For others, it could be vulnerability or authenticity. I would steer you away from broad-spectrum adjectives without defining how they show up specifically. **So get clear on specific adjectives and how they show up or manifest.** It's worth taking your time with curiosity.

Another way to find out your values is to ask yourself: What are my favorite characteristics about my current partner or closest friend? Maybe your closest friend or loved one that you admire has one or two things about them that are just pure gold. What's the adjective you would use to describe how they show up? How does that characteristic or description actually make you feel? I feel seen, heard, or acknowledged. I feel protected or adored. They understand me. Remember my dad at the Chinese buffet? This is one of a handful of people who I'd describe when doing this exercise for myself. It can be quite insightful to go through the list of close friends you've had in life and simply assign one good trait you thoroughly appreciated about them when they were in your life, regardless of who they are now.

Now, take all three processes that we just went through.

1. The painful voids that you've experienced, processed, and reverse-engineered to clarify the healthy characteristics you're after.

2. Unspoken red flags or rules in a close friendship.

3. What are your favorite characteristics in someone, and how do they make you feel?

(NOTE: It may be easier to go in reverse order 3,2,1 emotionally speaking to get in the vulnerable posture.)

Now look at the common denominators that have shown up there and pick your top 3 to 5 values on that list. How do these 3 to 5 core values show up for you in life?

Reflection Questions:

1. What are my roles?

_____

_____

_____

_____

2. What entities do I care about?

_____

_____

_____

_____

3. What are commonalities I enjoy with others?

4. What are some of your core values? (Three formulas to reveal your values; use all three.)

5. How does each value show up for you in action?

6. What does it tangibly cost you to live outside your values?

   _____

   _____

   _____

   _____

7. Can you imagine how fulfilling it will be to live with your values at the forefront of connections?

   _____

   _____

   _____

   _____

8. Once you get clear on what you value, ask yourself and your partner or friends these same questions you just answered if you'd like to go deep.

   _____

   _____

   _____

   _____

9. **If there are no shared values, are you willing to honor one another's values?**

   _____

   _____

   _____

   _____

   _____

10. **When you realize what it has cost you not to live in your values, are you willing to create intentionality around it in your relationships?**

    _____

    _____

    _____

    _____

    _____

As you begin to get clear on what your values are and how they show up in your life, you will look back at connections you previously cultivated and realize it was possibly your values that were in conflict.

Deep dive breakdown on values: it's easy to invite people into having your values, but authentic love pushes them to show up better in their own personal values. (Think about love languages. It's easier to love people in your love language, but it takes intentionality to love others in their love languages. **Apply this to values**.)

CHAPTER FOUR
CONFLICT MANAGEMENT

Fighting With Soft Gloves

It's never about the thing we're fighting over; it's likely about something deeper. We all know this deep down, yet pretend not to, and sometimes, we choose the wrong battle at the cost of feeling connected to our partner. Spoken with my dad's thickest, beautiful Middle Eastern accent, "it was the straw that broke the camel's back."

"You constantly throw your clothes on the floor as if I'm a maid here to serve your Highness."

"Might I make you a sandwich while the dishes are drying?"

"Ah, yes, the trash is overflowing, and our child needs their diaper changed."

What's there not to love? I can tell you, at the very least, this is no recipe for intimacy. Those sheets are cooling down after those comments. Most conflicts escalate to "Code Red" status but could have been resolved way earlier. Clearly set expectations, folks; it's incredible how valuable they are. When those expectations aren't met, or confusion arises, get curious without jumping to conclusions. Slow down, Batman. Introducing feedback into a relationship that's emotionally safe can save you hours and hours of unnecessary conflict.

I CAN'T SAY THIS ENOUGH. THE ANSWER TO CONFLICT IS TO DEPLOY CURIOSITY AND TRULY SEEK UNDERSTANDING. THEN, SHARE YOUR DATA, NARRATIVE AND ASK. You'll know what I mean as you read this chapter.

The secret sauce is that both parties want to be heard and understood during conflict, but it all starts with one thing—the narrative. This is the fear of previously experienced pain repeating itself in the present. The root lies beneath the symptom issue. It wasn't that he hadn't called me all day; he promised he would, and I know he gets busy, but I'm scared he's talking to someone else.

> *"The root lies beneath the symptom issue."*

Ah, there it is—the fear of being lied to or abandoned. That's the conflict beneath the surface. Most conflicts that arise are merely scratching another pain point from the past. If we're willing to pause before we even consider how to engage during a fight, there needs to be an awareness of what's leading someone to start it. You know, the classic dilemma of which came first, the chicken or the egg.

Keep this in mind: there is an inner child on the other side of the conversation steering their vehicle into the intersection, where anything could happen. It's also not your place to try and diagnose the trigger of the other person unless they've opened the door for feedback or an outside perspective. After you've taken ownership and things have been worked through, you can then ask, "Hey, can I share a perspective or submit a thought worth considering?" If you try to tell your partner why you think they're reacting at the beginning of a conversation, you will likely create unnecessary hurdles to overcome. **I am guilty of this.**

The truth is it takes one person inside a relationship to completely change the conflict dynamic. If you look at any sport, how you respond to what is given to you will change the game. Change your form, change your shot. I had to sit my two teenagers down and give them a solution to their ever-revolving sibling conflict. I took them to a park and stood them by a merry-go-round. I placed them on opposite sides of it. Whenever you experience conflict, and you show up poorly, you're both spinning that merry-go-round. Running to the victim card or accusing one another without taking ownership is messy, and the conflict gets bigger and harder to stop. I asked each one of them, "What's your contribution to this cycle? That is your 'response-ability.' What is yours to own? How are you helping create this painful event?" And eventually, they both got it. Now, when they're in conflict, and yes, I understand sometimes siblings fight, I ask them, "Are you done spinning?"(merry-go-round analogy.)

> "Running to the victim card or accusing one another without taking ownership is messy, and the conflict gets bigger and harder to stop."

I'm going to include a **sweet nugget of pure gold in this chapter—how to give a great apology**. Tell me how you would feel if someone were to apologize using some of the following statements:

- "I'm sorry you feel that way," or "I'm sorry you took it that way."

    (Translation: sounds like a *you* problem. Zero accountability for their contribution.)

- "You know I love you."

    (Translation: sidestepping or avoiding ownership is my preference, and I'd rather manipulate you, not apologize.)

- "Let's just move on," or "Can't we just forget it and move on?"

    (Translation: I don't want to deal with this now or ever, and I don't like the attention being on my mistakes.)

- "You are too sensitive. I didn't mean it like that."

    (Translation: I'd rather gaslight you and deflect by avoiding any responsibility or accountability.)

- Well, if you hadn't done that, then I wouldn't have acted this way."

    (I shouldn't have to translate by now, but we all realize these are victimized statements and garbage.)

- "Yeah, I'm sorry, but…"

    (Translation: apology null and void.)

(NOTE: These examples are from Angela Tobler and are a great example of how some people give shitty backhanded apologies. Not you, of course…)

Here's what you SHOULD DO. Take a deep breath. Pause until you can sincerely look them in the eye and slowly say the following:

"I apologize for raising my voice. I felt upset, and the story I created was that you didn't care. I realized my tone wasn't kind. I see that caused you to feel defensive and maybe even frustrated. I'll work on communicating without allowing my emotions to control my responses. Thank you for being gracious."

That's it.

Use this as a formula if you like, and make it your own for sincerity's sake. It'll do wonders.

- **State your actions like data.**
- **Elaborate on your internal story briefly without justification or excuses.**
- **Acknowledge your effects on them.**
- **Take ownership with a proactive agreement moving forward.**

Own your stuff and move on. Don't ask for forgiveness, give an explanation, or anything. Watch what happens. Some of you are too quick to own too much of other's actions, and you're enabling them. That needs to come back into a healthy balance. Some of you are way too fast to jump the gun and show your partner how they're wrong, justifying your actions and hurtful behavior. That, too, needs to come back into balance.

> *"Own your stuff and move on. Don't ask for forgiveness, give an explanation, or anything. Watch what happens."*

Those statements of, **"I'm sorry, your feelings got hurt." "I wouldn't do this if you didn't act like this; you made me do this." Those are a race-to-the-victim card and a self-fulfilling prophecy of duplicating pain over and over again.** There's ZERO ownership in them.

How you show up during conflict is up to you. That doesn't mean you act like a doormat or have a badge to act like a child ruled by their emotions. However, you can choose to create something you've never experienced by leaning in and showing up differently. Observe your nervous system reacting, notice what captures your attention, and be aware of the track playing in your mind as this conversation is unfolding.

Learn to observe yourself. They are not responsible for your emotions; yes, they have the ability to affect you, but you are responsible for how you respond. What you do with those emotions and how you unpack them is creating the experience.

When we establish the rules of engagement, we trust one another to honor the boundaries of our experiencing conflict together. **Conflict is one of the greatest gifts you'll ever experience.** *"That's dumb, Zach. Conflict sucks."* Yes, *and* **it reveals what's going on beneath the surface.** It's also a deeper invitation to connect as something that is disconnected internally is trying to reveal itself. It's like a boundary. When you establish a boundary, it's not for any reason other than intentional connection versus "stay out, you're not allowed" entry. No, it's actually a doorway that says, "I want to connect with you, but in this fashion." Conflict is a natural part of every relationship, but it can determine the outcome. **Choose your weapons carefully, for** *"The tongue holds the power of life and death."* This is about the need for fairness when conflict arises. Some would say never bring a gun to a knife fight, relationally speaking.

I was elated to attend my first sparring night at a Muay Thai gym. Sparring means lightly attacking with reserve and without landing heavy blows. It also means to engage in an argument that is not violent—in essence, **it's not high stakes**. At the Muay Thai gym, we warmed up and wore full, heavy gloves with shin pads. We paired off veterans against the newcomers on purpose, as the veterans knew the right pace for sparring. Well, let's just say you quickly learned where your skills stood. My coach at the time had a saying, **"Lessons not learned in blood are soon forgotten."** These words of wisdom were proven true at every session. I was paired with a sturdy, stocky, hairy ogre of a man who quickly taught me humility and self-awareness. We began exchanging combinations that included elbows, kicks, strikes, and throws. Due to my lack of sparring awareness, I landed blows slightly harder than he preferred. My opponent, the little giant, swiftly gave me feedback without any verbal warning by landing full kicks to my ribs. Heavy blows were exchanged in the name of self-preservation and ego. I was pretty sore for the next week, and to this day, I've never had such ugly bruises.

Truthfully, had this guy lowered his hands and given me any type of feedback, I would have paused and adjusted with no need for explanation. But instead, **like most conflicts, unnecessary pain was exchanged for the sake of preserving ego.**

(By the way, on the topic of ego, *Breaking Free from the Ego* by Trina Carroll-Houk is well worth the read.)

Too often, we do this with our partners. You need to learn how to verbally spar with your partner while honoring your truth doused in love. 90% of communication has nothing to do with the words, so look in the mirror and listen to your tone before engaging. Are your facial expressions, body language, and tonality warm and inviting into connection, or is it slightly asshole-ish in nature? If you take the time to do this well, you will learn what causes growth instead of causing hurtful, possibly permanent damage in each exchange. Conflict is a healthy part of relationships, and very few of us are well-versed in handling such a thing. It's lazy and ignorant to do otherwise. Sometimes, you might shut down, run away, or get crazy. This is a call to do better. For now, you are no longer ignorant. Some responses cause damage, and a lot of it.

> *"Are your facial expressions, body language, and tonality warm and inviting into connection, or is it slightly asshole-ish in nature?"*

If you subtract the weapons of warfare that reciprocate pain during conflict from your arsenal, it will lessen the damage experienced by you and your partner. Are you going to turn toward your partner in conflict or run away? Sure, take some time to cool down and collect your thoughts. Maybe even let your partner know this by setting an expectation to revisit the conversation at a later time. Remember this: **validating and collaborating will change everything if you take on this posture toward reconnecting.** (You can affirm or validate someone's experience without agreeing with it, they matter more than the differing perceptions.)

American psychologist Dr. John Gottman created the most accurate, provable, and well-documented content around committed relationships. The research is done for you; listen up. I will give you a dose of CliffsNotes to save you some time. His research shows that four things are sure KILLERS of any relationship. Before I tell you what they are, I have a challenge for you. Don't say to yourself, *Oh, my partner does this, and they do that.* Instead, ask how you can prove yourself guilty of any of them.

The "Four Horsemen" that destroy relationships are:

Criticism, Contempt, Defensiveness, **and** ***Stonewalling.***

They are predictors of doom, guaranteed to undermine any relationship. These four responses or actions, which emerge amidst conflict, are vigorously exposed, and clarification on how to resolve them is provided in the Gottman criteria. If you ask me, it's Relationship Intelligence 101 and just the beginning of creating intentional connections.

Question to consider:

Do you criticize or tear down your partner in any way? (Internally or externally)

_____

_____

_____

_____

At the end of the day, we all need to know how to navigate conflict in a sustainable way. If not, every relationship we acquire will reveal our lack of ability to do so, and we'll blame the world for our reality. I know guys that punish their wives with the silent treatment and are cold for days when they're pissed off. I hear of women who withhold intimacy to manipulate their husbands into submission. I see that both sexes demand immediate resolution with hostility. They call each other names, or they talk negatively about them to other people. Some victimize themselves fully committing to powerlessness or even their spouse's abusive behavior in some Stockholm syndrome type of dynamic. (Yes, physical entrapping abuse happens; I'm not negating the physical trap some have to escape.) Either posture can completely change the dynamic to a large extent when it comes to conflict. Let's try treating your partner/spouse like they're actually on your team instead of punishing them or victimizing them.

(Making others feel your pain doesn't remedy your own. Also, fixing others' pain prior to acknowledging your own doesn't solve anything. Both result in resentment.)

> **SIDE NOTE:** Your relationship is not a group project, so don't treat it like one. There's more harm than good by inviting others into your conflict with your partner. For some of you, everyone else is the problem, but you may not realize your contribution to those problems. If I told you those "four horsemen" are cancer to a relationship and a sure killer, and that you could avoid that cancer with a high survival rate, would you take the antidote?

Remember, you attract bees with honey, not vinegar.

Between using the conflict tool I'm about to describe and setting clear, measurable expectations with healthy boundaries, there is an 89.75 % chance a relationship will be widely successful so long as you both shall live. Seriously, if we taught young people how to identify their values and live from them along with these tools, **the divorce rate would drop so dramatically the entire country's culture would shift.**

Imagine not being able to connect with someone until you clear the air. You've got a lump in your throat and there's a proverbial elephant in the room that's stepping on your chest. You want to reconnect, but you're afraid of things getting intense or a misunderstanding taking place even worse. We call this a "fix a fight" type of tool in our house. It facilitates a conversation worth having that's clear, intentional, and effective.

FIX A FIGHT: This is a great simple template for an opportunity to have intentionally managed conflict. I'd really appreciate it if you shared any positive outcomes from these conflict remedies. (not sorry to ask for positive testimonials). Let's do a **#fixafight** as our tag wherever you post if you're feeling vulnerable.

FIX A FIGHT: DATA | NARRATIVES | OWNERSHIP | ASK

DATA: State the facts with no blaming, accusing, or shaming.

- Accusing or blaming games are a race to the victim card and it gives away your power. Instead, state facts as **DATA** points that involve no opinions or judgy statements.

NARRATIVES: (DON'T ACCUSE or BLAME)

- "You're a douche when we're at your parent's place."
- "Why are you being a schmuck?!"
- "It's amazing how you act when your friends are around (passive-aggressive classic)."

SAY THIS INSTEAD:

- "Your mood towards me seemed different when we were at your family's place. Are you doing ok?"
- "Is something bothering you that someone or I did?"
- "It's tough to experience the version of you I just did when your friends were around. (These are you inviting your partner into vulnerability.)"

OWNERSHIP: "I feel [X]." **Own your emotions**

- This allows you to feel seen and heard without blaming other people. Maybe even mention/own what it reminds you of in the past and the meaning you might assign to this experience that isn't theirs to own but how it impacts you.

DON'T SAY:

- "You made me feel [X]." That's dumb and victim-ish.

SAY THIS INSTEAD:

- "It hurt my feelings when you made that comment about me in front of your family. I felt demeaned and publicly shamed. It's something I never want to experience from you, of all people, and it reminds me of how my dad used to yell at us in public. He didn't care, and deep down, I can't imagine ever feeling that way again by someone I love."

- o **"I could have done [XYZ] better or differently."** Ownership is disarming and inviting further into vulnerability and ownership on their end.
- "If I was being too playful or did something that made you feel embarrassed, I'm open to discussing that. Up until now, I haven't made it clear that I'm not ok with being spoken to like that, not even as a joke."

ASK: Make a sincere request clearly known

- It can be denied, FYI, so this may be an opportunity for a personal boundary to be communicated instead or for you to understand what your partner is not willing to change.

SAY THIS:

- "If you're bothered by something, please come to me in private instead of making fun of me."
- "I love you being playful with me, but I can't tolerate being put down in any way. That's a turn-off for me and extremely hurtful. I'd ask you not to cross that bridge again, as how we interact in friend/family settings means a lot to me."

DO THIS:

- **Some type of physical contact.** Hugging it out, holding hands, but make it last for 30 seconds. No choking, lol. This might feel uncomfortable as our inclination is to recluse and not reconnect, but it's really helpful when we do.

DATA - NARRATIVES - OWNERSHIP - ASK

Use this formula; it'll serve you in the future. Remember this as a baseline for simple conflict resolution in all connections. If you're feeling edgy and vulnerable, upload a video of how it worked for you and tag us in your conflict resolution. The good, bad, and ugly… that's the fertilizer of life. **#fixafight.**

When you sense a potential blowup is on the horizon, yank the emotional wheel away from the cliff and hit the brakes. Hey, let's push pause. Let's get intentional before this cliff dive takes place, and unnecessary damage happens. It's completely avoidable moving forward. Use the FIX A FIGHT or even just this posture around conflict. This template, when used in conversation, works in any conflict when used as an outline.

> **Nuggets to snack on:** Just because you think a thought doesn't make it true. We need to feed our brains new information, creating new pathways for neurons. Otherwise, your BS narrative stays on repeat. Watching *Titanic* once was enough for a lifetime. The boat sinks; don't recreate unnecessary drama. Your brain equates safety with repetition, so be aware of that. Read that again: scientifically proven, your brain tricks you into creating its version of safety. I'm not telling you to gaslight yourself, but I am reminding you of the power of a false narrative. **Unhealed narratives will trick you into repeating painful emotional cycles.** What has always been your experience

> doesn't have to remain so. Remember, the majority of communication is not about the words you use. It's about your posture, attitude, and tone.

Reflection Questions:

1. What area of conflict management could you grow in?

   _____
   _____
   _____
   _____
   _____

2. Do you criticize or tear down your partner in any way? (Internally or externally.)

   _____
   _____
   _____
   _____
   _____

3. Do you find yourself feeling contempt for your partner?

_____
_____
_____
_____

4. Are you aware your contempt shows in some capacity?

_____
_____
_____
_____

5. Do you stonewall in any form?

_____
_____
_____
_____

6. Is resentment forming? If so, what do you perceive the cause is?

   _____

   _____

   _____

   _____

7. How well do you process your trigger before engaging in conflict?

   _____

   _____

   _____

   _____

8. How do you initially respond to conflict?

   _____

   _____

   _____

   _____

9. Do you create conflict when a soft approach or curious question would change everything?

_____

_____

_____

10. Do you pay attention to the internal dialog you have with yourself before reacting?

_____

_____

_____

11. What model of conflict management did you watch growing up?

_____

_____

_____

12. How does that model recreate itself in your connections today?

_____

_____

_____

_____

13. What toxic responses or reactions do you bring to conflicts?

_____

_____

_____

_____

14. If connection was a currency, how much are these toxic traits costing you?

_____

_____

_____

_____

15. How could you confront your partner in a healthy, safe and inviting way?

_____

_____

_____

_____

_____

PS. For those who are crazy brave, invite feedback from someone you love and trust into these questions.

An entire relationship can shift in dynamics simply because one partner decides to grow. I've single-handedly witnessed partnerships change time and again, simply because one party decided to start showing up differently. They shifted their focus from their partner's flaws to their own need for growth. Instead of casting blame or accusations on their partner for everything that goes wrong in the relationship, they looked in the mirror and began to take ownership of how they showed up. (I'm not condoning one-sided relationships where one partner refuses to ever take ownership or grow.) If two people genuinely want to grow their connection with one another, this approach is a great tool to have in their relational toolkit. Regardless, this skill can be applied to every connection you wish to maintain in your life.

If couples would grasp the idea that success lies on the other side of both individuals committing to show up better, their relationship would transform almost immediately. It's funny; as I write this, I'm reminded of Forrest Gump leaning against his loyal friend Bubba in the midst of war so they don't sleep in the mud. **Once both individuals in a relationship begin to take ownership, conflicts or problems within that relationship become an "us versus the issue," not "you versus me."**

This is the posture of what we call power couples, alignment not just in goals but in posture alongside one another. I mention this because, either way, whether you stay in the relationship or leave, you're going to have to face your issues eventually. And there's no better time to do that than when you're in a relationship, getting triggered constantly, as that's what relationships do—they reveal what's inside you. I'm not a proponent of making things work at all costs, nor do I wish divorce on anyone. However, I am a huge believer and supporter of pursuing growth at all costs, regardless of the relationship's outcome. Ownership will become the new lens through which you view the creation of the relational experience you desire. Remember, conflict reveals beliefs and narratives. **The more we can learn how to navigate THROUGH conflict, the more we will learn it is working only in our favor.**

> *"I am a huge believer and supporter of pursuing growth at all costs, regardless of the relationship's outcome. Ownership will become the new lens through which you view the creation of the relationship experience you desire."*

CHAPTER FIVE

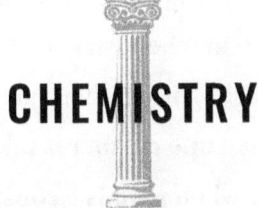

CHEMISTRY

Ya Feel Me? (Insert Side Eye)

His pursuit of her involves ignoring her, and for reasons that defy logic, she'll chase him down, wondering, "Why doesn't he like me? I'll show him what he's missing out on." Ironically, if he gives her too much attention, she'll run away, thinking, "He must not have much going for him if he's so readily available for me." This is a classic example of toxic chemistry that reinforces the dysfunctional patterns normalized in our culture. It merely reflects the childhood model and perpetuates unhealthy connections into adulthood. Toxic behavior is often mistaken for chemistry, feeding into a pattern that sustains emotional addiction. (Yes, this idea around childhood models appears in marriage as well as dating, albeit less subtly in new connections.)

We could substitute the words "attraction" and "chemistry" for a moment of enlightenment. Men and women view attraction through different lenses. It's universally acknowledged that there are different levels of attraction. You might find the bartender pouring a drink or a firefighter attractive, but it doesn't necessarily mean much. The key is to acknowledge attraction and build upon it. It's interesting how people often lose weight after breakups and gain weight when they enter relationships, easing off the behaviors that initially bring attraction into the relationship. They stop buying flowers, writing love notes, and acknowledging the little things. Connective tissue in chemistry is formed when two parties appreciate each other, highlighting their greatness and individuality. **Attraction diminishes when one partner is taken for granted, when one is overly self-absorbed, or when pain is a constant experience.**

There are people in your life with whom you can communicate without words. When something happens, all it takes is a look, and you're both on the same page. It's often laughably accurate. This dynamic brings a lot of laughter into your life and moments worth remembering. Playfulness and the ability to emotionally connect are incredibly important. It doesn't take a rocket scientist to notice couples who are in survival mode and can barely tolerate each other's presence. A friendship or connection without chemistry is almost transactional, or as some might call it, an arrangement. Don't get me wrong, arrangements can work, especially when chosen intentionally, as some indeed are. Read between the lines here: they'll function for survival, maybe even help you through a few decades. Like a terrible performance by your uncle at a family reunion karaoke, you wish that song would end.

Personalities don't have to match for there to be chemistry. In fact, he could be as legitimately dry as a British sitcom, and she could have the wit of the Three Stooges, but they understand and appreciate each other. That's the key: understanding each other. Have you ever caught yourself thinking, "Yeah, he or she just gets me," and it's nice to have that? **Emotional connections cultivated in friendship, intimate trust, and**

meaningful conversations create a baseline for incredible chemistry. And when you have incredible chemistry, there's a chance your sexual connection will be top-shelf, crème de la crème, exactly what you deserve.

You know that couple who seems to love fighting? It's almost as if they don't know how to handle peace without creating chaos, believing they must push each other away before pulling closer again. That's massively unhealthy, and their brains are recreating trauma scenarios to feel "safe." **Remember, the brain equates repetition with safety.**

There may be some people who bring calmness or peace, and maybe you're not used to feeling this way. Perhaps your brain prefers the nervous, neurotic unpredictability and toxicity, mistakenly identified as chemistry. Yes, that's a problem, and it's not something to brag about anymore. Couples out there who play fight all the time or create conflict to feel connected—you know who you are. Consider this an opportunity to redefine healthy chemistry for yourselves.

The point I'm trying to make about chemistry is that you need it. It takes only five minutes to find 100 ways to maintain chemistry in a relationship, and most of them require intentionality. Men, if you want her to feel aroused, know that chemistry is created long before the bedroom. It begins with you creating a safe environment for her to be vulnerable and stay in her feminine essence. Women, to cultivate chemistry with your man, tell him what you like about him and do playful things with him. You can be playful and join him without stepping into your masculine. The bedroom only reveals the depth of intimate knowledge you have of each other emotionally. Otherwise, it's merely a transactional exchange and, at best, unsustainable. The bedroom reveals so much about a couple that one could reverse engineer most of their relationship by observing how they engage sexually, but that's not the focus of this discussion.

I recall watching couples in a dance competition on TV, and it was apparent who was mustering up the strength to perform and who was authentically present in the moment. The simplicity of getting along in the small moments—being playful, challenging each other to reach their potential—is crucial. It's what will carry you through a multitude of life experiences: the ability to laugh after crying your eyes out, the flirting, the unique language you share. Just being with someone amidst chaos, unexpected painful moments, or having them close to celebrate victories is life-changing.

> **Push pause:** What's the one thing you're afraid of bringing up that will destroy the mood? What's one unresolved and open-ended thing that your partner keeps bringing up? **That topic will likely harm your relationship and act as a "chemistry" killer, as it introduces elements that undermine emotional safety.**

If you lack chemistry even in a friendship, chances are it's as dry as the Phoenix heat, and the connection is likely on borrowed time. Chemistry isn't the sole deciding factor, but it's certainly one of the four pillars that can render a relationship either mediocre or beautiful. Do you resonate with someone? Is there a sense of cohesiveness? Do you blend well in each other's presence?

Imagine your best friend introduces you to someone, and after interacting, you both walk away. Deep down, you know you don't like this person, and even if you can't pinpoint why, it's clear they're not on your wavelength. We can discern whether we have chemistry with someone, and it's unhealthy to base an entire relationship on what is essentially a one-legged table, yet people do it all the time, often citing exceptional sexual chemistry as justification. But is the person emotionally safe and trustworthy? Remember, like a free diver running out of air, you'll eventually need to surface and face reality. Chemistry should be a gently nurtured flame, not an unsustainable chemical explosion.

> *"We can discern whether we have chemistry with someone. However, it's unhealthy to base an entire relationship on what is essentially a one-legged table. Yet, people do it all the time, often citing exceptional sexual chemistry as justification."*

If I had to softly redefine the concept of chemistry, I'd say it's the outcome of collaborative effort towards building an emotional connection, thriving together in life, and genuinely supporting each other emotionally and physically. Pursuing your partner in the ways you always have once you've been together for a while is like letting off the gas. **You *won* them, *keep* them by doing the things that attracted them to you initially and stay creative by sowing new seeds of love. You'll be surprised at what sprouts up in the garden of their heart.**

I can't tell you what creates chemistry between you and your partner. Maybe it's thoughtfulness in action, or it could be the way your partner looks at you across the room in a moment. Maybe they write you notes to remind you they care. It's typically the little things I've found to create chemistry in couples, no matter what.

I can tell you, though, a few things that will absolutely destroy *chemistry* in a heartbeat: **criticism, unprocessed pain,** and **repetitive conflict**. Criticism and harsh, repetitive conflicts are withdrawals from your energetic relational bank account. Not only do you need to make more deposits into your partner's heart, but criticism and intense conflicts also deplete our emotional accounts significantly. I see many couples connect well, but they forget that you need five positive interactions for every one negative interaction.

Remember this if you want to create incredible chemistry.

Reflection Questions:

Look at your last few romantic connections or your current one.

1. **Is chemistry in your relationships based upon healthy, safe, inviting, playful behavior? Or is it based on toxic behaviors that induce repetition of childhood traumas?**

    _____

    _____

    _____

    _____

    _____

    _____

2. What was the chemistry based upon?

_____

_____

_____

_____

_____

_____

3. How would you rate your chemistry on a scale of 1-10? (No 7s allowed.)

_____

_____

_____

_____

_____

_____

4. Was/Is chemistry the only connecting point?

   _____
   _____
   _____
   _____
   _____
   _____

5. What's the lack of chemistry costing you in feeling connected?

   _____
   _____
   _____
   _____
   _____
   _____

6. Is it under or over-emphasized in your relationships? Are you willing and able to commit to chemistry being a priority in your relationship?

_____

_____

_____

_____

_____

_____

7. What's it going to take to get that chemistry wheel turning in the right direction?

_____

_____

_____

_____

_____

_____

CHAPTER SIX

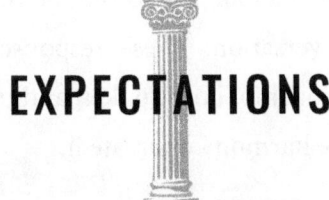

EXPECTATIONS

Bids, Booty Calls and Boundaries (#expectations)

I should consider dedicating an entire chapter to the idea of wooing our partners and the importance of responding to them authentically, but instead, I'll explain why failing to do so is a deal-breaker for two reasons. If you don't respond to them at all, it **will build up resentment in your partner.** If you respond to them merely to please your partner and not authentically, you'll ignite a long fuse that, over years, **reveals a preference for prioritizing others' needs over your own and mislabeling it as love.** This eventually leads to a breakdown.

Let's talk about intimacy. You've made it this far; what did you expect? If you were to honestly describe your sex life with your partner (or a previous one if you're single), there's a high chance it would offer a snapshot of your relationship. Now, if the reviews were to provide an all-encompassing description of the emotional connectivity points regarding your intimacy, what would they say?

What is the baseline for how you and your partner respond to each other's bids? (Bids are any form of reaching out to one another to gain attention or connection.) It could be something small, like pointing out a bird, a hand grab, or even a look across the room. It could be formalized into a request or conversation. These responses create much of the dynamics in your relationship, both spoken and unspoken. It's the small things that can spoil the harmony or create it.

Reflect on how bids manifest in your relationship from both sides. Consider each other's responses. We are vulnerable creatures, perhaps more than we realize, especially in terms of the unspoken dynamics in a relationship. If your partner constantly flirts with you and you respond positively half the time, they have a 50/50 positive to negative bid ratio. If you are ignored by your partner or ridiculed 2 out of 3 times, you might experience a 66% negative interaction rate and wonder where feelings of resentment stem from. I guarantee you haven't measured bids in your relationship. Don't panic, but understand that this dynamic either contributes to a full love tank or to a deficiency in the relationship. Do you feel emotionally connected in all aspects? Is the intimacy what you desire?

> *"We are vulnerable creatures, perhaps more than we realize, especially to the unspoken dynamics in a relationship."*

Boundaries reveal as much about the person setting them as they do about how others respond. If I say, "Having lunch with your parents no longer works for me. It's really taxing emotionally, but I'm open to connecting with them, just less frequently," that's a straightforward, unapologetic boundary, indicative of my personality and who I am as a person.

However, if I say, "Please don't be mad at me. I really love spending time with you and your family. I know they're super important to you, and it's nice that we get to see them every week. I don't want to hurt their feelings or yours, but can I skip this week? You can totally go without me. It's just that I'm really tired and don't have it in me," people who prefer direct communication might find all the fluff and lack of directness in this example frustrating. Meanwhile, those who prioritize others' feelings over their own might think this sounds about right or perhaps even feel it wasn't considerate enough.

It's not about right vs. wrong—it's more about revealing your emotional makeup in how you go about setting boundaries or making bids to your partner. It's about managing your own needs with self-love and honoring the expectations you've set with others. Some of you are so self centered and need to consider others more often. Some of you need to stop focusing on others' needs and fill your own tank first. Both need to come into balance and can learn something from the other.

Maybe you have a partner who sets asshole-ish boundaries. For example, they might say, "Hey, I'm not going to lunch this week with your parents. They suck the soul out of me, and I'm over it. Do whatever you want." This approach reveals a lot, much of which shouldn't need to be spelled out, but it's worth mentioning this: adopting a "my way or the highway" attitude without offering any explanation is rather inconsiderate. Don't get me wrong, "no thank you" is a complete sentence, and it's perfectly acceptable. However, it's also okay to give your partner some insight into your reasons.

> **Gold nugget:** Compromise should not replace boundaries. On the other hand, co-creation is a better approach.

As you grow in self-awareness and emotional intelligence, you'll discover tools you can use to maintain healthy self-love. Boundaries are only as effective as their enforcement. Therefore, it's futile to establish and communicate a boundary if there are no consequences for its violation. There are thousands of simple boundary outlines online and some incredible books that reveal both the need for and how to apply them. While I'm not here to teach you how to do that, I am here to tell you it's very important and effective. At their core, boundaries are an invitation to a safe connection. I once heard a guru say, "Walls keep everyone out, but boundaries teach people where the door is. I want to connect with you, but [XYZ] cannot continue to happen. Otherwise, this doesn't work for me. Here's what I'm willing to do that works for me."

Setting boundaries is not about constant threats or manipulative tactics; it should be clear and definable. **When done correctly and respected by the other party involved, it creates trust and safety.** Well-established boundaries are attractive and reveal much about one another and the type of connection being cultivated. People's responses to a "no" or to boundaries being set reveal a lot about them, about you, and about your relationship dynamic.

Question to ask:

1. Are you fluent in setting/managing boundaries?

_____

_____

_____

_____

One thing that makes me laugh: when people advise others to not have expectations, suggesting this will prevent disappointment. This advice is far from wise. When people are consistently present in your life, communicating clear expectations in some form is essential.

It's time to clarify what your expectations are for this relationship, your partner, and yourself if you plan to stay. Take out your yellow steno pad and write down the unmet spoken expectations and the expectations that have been met for which you're grateful. Now, let's be brutally honest and identify the expectations that are unspoken and underlying in your heart. Maybe you've never acknowledged being disappointed about certain things or realized that they mattered to you. However, simply acknowledging those unmet expectations can save you and your partner from resentment if you're staying in connection. If you recall from earlier in the book, resentment is one of the pillars and fatal blows to a relationship. Addressing this can also save you from massive amounts of conflict.

A childhood friend of mine recently re-entered my life after 25 years. His wife is a full-time homemaker, while he works three jobs. He told me, "Zach, I realized I needed to step up more after seeing her get overwhelmed with the little things that needed to get done, like the dishes every night, regardless of whether she or I cooked. I consciously made a commitment to handle them. No matter what meal she made, it was now my job every day to ensure they were done. If I missed a day, I felt like I was letting her down. Handling things around the house is the absolute least I can do, as she's giving so much of herself to our kids. I've come to realize it's not about the dishes. It's about her knowing I'm right here with her, and it's the little things that show we're in this together." He aimed to set an expectation she could trust and rely on.

Now, before you roll your eyes, consider that there are many things in our own households that trigger us, revealing that we actually feel taken for granted. This breeds resentment and despair, only to be expressed indirectly towards our partner and ourselves, maybe even our children. **Acknowledgment creates an opportunity for gratitude. Also, ignoring our partner's bids for connection can lead to resentment, which is the ultimate relationship killer.**

Mediators witness everything in divorce cases; in fact, it's downright wildly entertaining to listen to them share war stories about the depths of human ugliness. Amid the ending of a relationship, a highly skilled mediator shared with me a revelation she had while sitting across from a volatile couple. If spouses were to set pre-mediated expectations with one another regarding as many scenarios as they could think of together, they would be surprised at how well-insulated their relationships would become. The frustrations and accusations that emerge during mediations often stem from mismanaged expectations, resentments, and unspoken wounds—all sadly byproducts of a lack of intentionality and honest communication. It's interesting to hear someone who witnesses the unraveling of marriages on a daily basis share a perspective.

Question for you: Have you made your expectations clear? Is your partner absolutely clear on those expectations, both minor and significant? Once you've clarified your expectations, it's time to discuss them with your partner and assess expectations from both sides. When a couple takes the time to clarify their expectations and manage them—because as time goes on and life happens, expectations need to be managed proactively—it can make a significant difference in the relationship's outcome. I know couples who schedule time alone and date nights on their calendars. Hey, if you don't get intentional about it, it'll never happen. So, kudos to them. For some reason, our culture becomes obsessed and distracted by gender roles and symptomatic issues that would cease to exist if couples got clear on their expectations of one another. By the way, this is not an opportunity to create a hostage negotiation or make demands. It's simply to say, "This is what I'm expecting of you based on what you've said; this is what I'm expecting of the experience I want to create within our relationship. What are yours?"

> *"When a couple takes the time to clarify their expectations and manage them—because as time goes on and life happens, expectations need to be managed proactively—it can make a significant difference in the relationship's outcome."*

> **Side note:** if there is something you need in your relationship that you're not getting or a need that's not being met, you need to ask yourself, have I truly clearly communicated measurable actions that I'd like my partner to take?

Men, I need to have a serious conversation with you for a moment. If you interact with your partner to merely get your physical needs met, the timer has begun. Thinking you're entitled to sex is an unhealthy mindset, and frankly, it's astonishing to hear. There's a healthier way to have your needs met, and I'm here to guide you toward experiencing it. Treating sex with your partner as if it's a piggy bank where you make emotional deposits, and then feeling upset when she doesn't reciprocate is not the way to go. You're part of that exchange, so it's your responsibility to make her feel loved and safe enough to cultivate intimacy with you. Ask yourself: Are you emotionally manipulative or controlling? Are you neglecting your physical health or not wooing her like you did in the beginning? Are you acting like a doormat? Neither approach leads to intimacy. Embrace your masculine energy and stop looking for transactional interactions. Don't feel entitled to intimacy; instead, ask her what makes her feel safe, loved, and pursued. She's with you for a reason—keep adding to that list and pursue her passionately. Unravel her heart with every action you take, and she'll blossom like a sun-gazing wildflower.

If she no longer wants to have sex and you're clueless as to why, ask yourself: *How am I showing up for her?* Do you contribute around the house or with the kids? Do you do everything and expect nothing from her, ironically resenting her, when in reality, you're frustrated with yourself for creating this dynamic? When you do the dishes, do you expect sex in return? Take a moment to reflect on how transactional your perspective might be. What does it look like to fill her love tank? How do you maintain your integrity while pursuing her without self-deprecation? Are you aware of what being in your authentic masculine energy entails? What toxic behaviors do you introduce into your sex life?

Ladies, do you use sex as leverage? Do you engage in it just to keep him happy? Do you approach him with vulnerable honesty about how you want your heart to be pursued? Is your conversation with your partner approached with care or criticism? While we all surely love feedback, inviting your partner into connection with authenticity is truly appealing. Sex reveals so much about a couple; it's enlightening when both partners are honest about their dynamics. The truth is it often uncovers a lot of emotional pain, trauma, or beliefs, which can be daunting. What brings out your feminine side? What encourages you to embrace your masculine energy? What aspects of your relationship are reflected in your sex life?

Back to both of you. Ask yourself: *Am I willing to accept what I'm getting without anything changing and simply grieve the loss of that need while I'm in the relationship?* I recently had a couple come to me, and during our conversation, she said, "I think I'm just willing to let go of certain desires that I'm never going to experience within this relationship." I could see both resolve and disappointment cross her face. You may not have your need met, or it might not be fulfilled in the way you desire within this relationship.

Perhaps you'd prefer to maintain the relationship you have, valuing what you *do* receive over the risk of being without this person. Maybe there are things your heart can't bear to go without, however painful it may be to leave the relationship. Only you have the true answer.

Question to ask:

1. Do you take ownership of managing and setting clear expectations?

___

___

___

___

___

___

2. How well do you respond when someone sets a boundary with you?

___

___

___

___

___

___

3. How would you rate your tendency to please others on a scale from 1 to 10? For example, can you sit with uncomfortable emotions, or do you feel the need to alleviate such feelings for others and yourself?

_____

_____

_____

_____

_____

4. Do you leverage something your partner desires, such as sex, money, or attention, to experience you? (For example, do you justify manipulative behavior as a means of exchange?)

_____

_____

_____

_____

_____

5. Is your sex life interactive emotionally and intimately, or is it transactional?

6. Describe your love life with a movie quote or title. (For example, *Gone with the Wind* or *Gone in 60 Seconds*.)

7. What title would you love it to be?

_____

_____

_____

_____

_____

8. When you share your feelings, does your partner shut you down?

_____

_____

_____

_____

_____

9. Do you acknowledge your partner when they communicate a bid?

_____

_____

_____

_____

10. Are you and your partner happy with your sex life?

_____

_____

_____

_____

11. Is your sex life a "make or break" for one of you?

_____

_____

_____

_____

12. Do YOU understand what healthy boundaries look like?

_____

_____

_____

_____

13. What are you afraid of when it comes to boundaries? Are you willing and able to say no?

14. Are there clearly set expectations on both sides of the relationship? Are you willing to audit them together?

15. Are we happy with how you both communicate and make bids for physical and emotional connection?

16. Are you both content with each other's responses?

17. What does physical intimacy reveal about your emotional connection to one another?

18. Do you take ownership of managing and setting clear expectations?

_____
_____
_____
_____

19. How do you respond when expectations that were clearly set are not met?

_____
_____
_____
_____

20. Is there an opportunity for growth in your relationship around expectations?

_____
_____
_____
_____

SECTION 3
EXIT

"You can skip this part if you're happily married. Definitely read chapter 9."

CHAPTER SEVEN
What if I'm Done?

You might not relate to this part; in fact, some of it is embarrassing in hindsight, but it reveals what's in a lot of us. I waited too long to come up for air. My heart had negotiated with its own fears and pain for years without realizing what was happening. There are two extremes that occur when someone is in a relationship and the end is possibly near. They seek advice not from someone who has what they want, but instead, they listen to advice that only affirms their shame, fear, and obligations. Sitting in front of friend after friend, negotiating for my own heart without knowing they were reflecting my own beliefs.

Divorce is considered wrong at all costs, and "God hates divorce," which internally feels like *God hates you for this.* Pastors pleaded with me, asking if there was any way to make it work. What is everyone's obsession with keeping people married at all costs in the name of religion? Looking back, it's like I was pleading and negotiating with myself, trying to figure out what judgment I harbored towards myself if I followed through with ending my relationship. I was deeply afraid of God's judgment, which was partially true because of my upbringing. What would happen to my faith if I was willing to "go against the pastor's advice"? Just typing this makes me nauseous at how controlling and destructive the projections we put onto God are, taught by our parents and "spiritual leaders."

> *"Looking back, it's like I was pleading and negotiating with myself, trying to figure out what judgment I harbored towards myself if I followed through with ending my relationship."*

If you're in a religious upbringing or mindset, I want you to know YOU matter more to God than your marital experience. I don't care who this offends. If your faith is based on this, it's shifting in your favor. Thinking you "staying married" somehow undoes your faith means it was faith in you, not Him. I was outsourcing my self-love, hoping for one person to ask me, "Hey, if you're done, man, I have your back. I'm right here, no matter what. You matter to me more than your relationship status." Seriously, I know a guy who wrote an entire book against this paradigm. It's a brilliant case for divorce. That's right, there's a time and a place to end a relationship. How you go about that ending is utterly up to you. Remember this: no healthy relationship is a group project. When you invite multiple people's opinions into a relationship, it's a recipe for disaster, a decision for grown adults to make on their own.

The next time someone tells you they're thinking of leaving their marriage or ending the relationship, weigh your words carefully and invite them to be clear on how you can support them lovingly through this. When someone's heart is hurting, believe them. I've never been so "gaslit" in my life—except by myself. People will only treat you to the level you've trained them to. You don't need anyone's approval to make decisions. In fact, making decisions is a clear sign of self-leadership. You've likely outsourced your self-trust, and now it's come to a head after years of accumulated pain. This isn't to say you're a victim, but you're finally realizing you can't keep demeaning yourself by staying in a relationship that no longer serves your highest authentic direction. If you're deciding to stay in the connection, that's great. I salute you with sincere support. Double down and go for it, but don't lie to yourself about why you're staying or if that motivation needs to be examined. The best advice in this scenario is to pause and get clear on where you're at and what your heart needs.

"I feel like I'm sitting in a boat, and I don't want to be here anymore. I want to get out of this damn boat," I said to my life coach. I had just found out that my girlfriend had slept with her ex. Ironically, this was my first real relationship after my divorce.

He said, "Zach, you're allowed to get out of the boat. You get to do whatever you want to do. You get to decide if you want to forgive her and stay in the relationship or if it's time to move on."

It was interesting because, at that very moment, it felt like the huge pressure to stay was gone. It's funny how everything changes when you permit yourself to do something for the first time.

For many reasons, probably due to the model of love I grew up watching, I had this weird obligation and shame reflex that says, at all costs, you make your relationship work. If you love someone and you're committed to them, you figure out a way, no matter the cost, even to yourself. What I didn't realize at that moment was that the fear of being alone was driving me to constantly try to make things work in whatever relationship I was in. **In reality, I was teaching my partner to abandon me by abandoning myself first. Thus, I was only able to attract partners who would reaffirm my wounds.** There is a profound teaching: the unhealed pain within you will find a way to get your attention until you fully acknowledge it, sit with it, and hear its message until you heal it.

> *"If you love someone and you're committed to them, you figure out a way, no matter the cost, even to yourself. What I didn't realize at that moment was that the fear of being alone was driving me to constantly try to make things work in whatever relationship I was in."*

It would be years before I realized what wounds were trying to show themselves to me, but I would once again mute the microphone. My pursuit of that partner would take quite a timeline of connecting and disconnecting before the acknowledgment of the reality that the relationship needed to end.

So, you're leaving or heavily considering it. Now what? If you're looking to navigate through a necessary separation of any kind, you should probably read this section twice. I fully expect you to ignore some of what I'm telling you and possibly have to learn from your own pain. This is for those who don't need to learn the hard way. Some of us never touched the red burner on the stove. Wisdom heeds the warnings provided by the pain of others. And yes, I swear, my little sister blatantly ignored my mother. I'll never forget that scream as she decided to fully place her hand on the stove's red-hot burner. (Some of you might be too young to remember the cigarette lighter in cars, but I'll be damned if we didn't all touch that thing at some point).

Imagine hiking up Mount Everest and, along the way, stepping over hundreds of dead bodies, only to focus on your goal of reaching the summit. Yes, this actually happens on a weekly basis. Can you imagine the thoughts crossing your mind as you walk past half-buried, frozen bodies who thought they had the trek all figured out, just like you? Those dead bodies represent people who have encountered a level of failure and pain you haven't yet experienced. I'm sure if given the chance, those who failed the climb would have a few words of wisdom to share.

In the midst of leaving a relationship, no matter what, you're bound to make some mistakes and relive old patterns of your own. This is an opportunity to minimize the collateral damage when you leave, both in your life and in the lives of others. You might be thinking, *Oh, I just need to get out of here and sow my royal oats. I'll get fit and sexy, maybe even have a glow-up. That'll show them what they're missing out on. I'll become super successful, so I never experience this pain again.* Or my favorite new inner vow: *Never let someone in again.* **All of it is complete nonsense.** We all know what's happening. When you change your profile picture and start posting your own narrative on social media, everyone knows what's going on. Regardless of whether you're right or validated in your story, shut it all down. Get quiet and do your freaking inner work. Go process the season you just created in your life. Otherwise, you'll find yourself back here, feeling the same way, in no time.

You don't have to spend more than 30 seconds online to encounter pop psychology terms like self-love, narcissists, empathy, etc. Regardless of how your ex treated you, what they did, how terrible of a villain they are, or maybe they're just not a good fit for you, the time to look everywhere else is over. **This is about you and you alone.** The quick fixes that people run to are sex, fitness, partying, or isolation. It's all fake self-love nonsense that produces no real healing or actual growth.

Self-love starts with acknowledging what's truly going on inside and processing the meanings we have assigned to it. Yes, we are meaning-assigning machines. We look at every event, every conflict, every conversation, and assign a meaning to it. You did, too; just think about your last breakup and listen to the things your brain whispered to you internally. Ironically, scientists have proven that our subconscious holds on to the meaning of the event, the meaning we assign to the pain, the narrative behind what they did to us, or what we experienced, not just the actual event itself.

> *"Self-love starts with acknowledging what's truly going on inside and processing the meanings we have assigned to it... We look at every event, every conflict, every conversation, and assign a meaning to it."*

I think they could write a hundred books on grief, and we'd still not cover all of how to do it well. In our culture, it's something you rarely hear taught. And that is grieving: the power of it, the necessity of it, and, funnily enough, the lack of its healthy expression in our lives. If and when your relationship ends, I want you to know that one of the best gifts you can give to yourself is the permission to grieve. You see, grief is a funny thing. It usually hits at the most inconvenient moments in life. You could be in the midst of a conversation, watching a movie, or simply at work, and that emotion, that visual aid comes to mind, and all of a sudden, you feel these intense feelings, and you think, *No, not now, later.* Don't schedule grief; honor it, and feel it fully when it comes up; you'll thank yourself later.

You might reach for a hand to comfort you or a drink to push away the emotion when, in fact, what's trying to surface is actually trying to serve you. Apologies for the visual in advance, but imagine an emotional "zit," if you will, trying to release toxins of trauma from your actual nervous system. If you're reading this, you're probably aware of all the books teaching that trauma is trapped in the body. Emotions are stored in our nervous system, where expressed grief grants the permission to release. This relationship, friendship, and connection need to be grieved.

There are a thousand different ways to pursue healing properly in your life, but this book is definitely here to emphasize the need for it. Imagine an airport runway in your heart and it's covered full of planes. In order for something new and fulfilling to land on that runway, you must first clear the pathway. This means you have the opportunity to forgive yourself first and the painful beliefs that led you to the relationship or kept you in it. It means stepping into the pain and feeling it fully without making it your identity. Remember, your response to pain determines your trajectory.

> *"This means you have the opportunity to forgive yourself first and the painful beliefs that led you to the relationship or kept you in it."*

It's time to choose your counsel wisely.

My hope is that you come to whatever conclusion you decide regarding the relationship on your own terms before chewing on the tabloid opinions of your friends—no offense. Kingdoms rise and fall following poor advice and unsound wisdom. If someone hasn't successfully navigated where you want to go, take it with a grain of salt. I'm not saying people without children can't give good parenting advice. However, I graciously hesitate to accept it at face value. What is valuable is learning from others' mistakes.

The same goes for ending relationships. We all have those friends who seem to have it all figured out and have an opinion on every aspect of life. Choose wisely who you surround yourself with. Men and women, for different reasons, avoid looking in the mirror with proactive accountability. People stubbornly avoid asking themselves, *How did I help create this scenario?* These are general tendencies, but we tend to isolate and not seek outside perspective until the relationship has actually reached its end, and by then, it's too late. Some place too much weight on their friends' opinions and complain about their partner until they've been convinced it's over. Maybe you're not like them, and you let your pain build up like an internal geyser, deciding to finally take action only when your heart can take no more.

> *"Men and women, for different reasons, avoid looking in the mirror with proactive accountability. People stubbornly avoid asking themselves, 'How did I help create this scenario?'"*

You might handle your exit with the ease and grace of a Russian ballet dancer, but I did not. It's one of the seasons of my life I wish I had handled better. Unfortunately, in survival mode, we do things without realizing the collateral damage that could follow. This damage might affect not just others involved but ourselves in the future as well. There's wisdom in a multitude of wise counsel—the keyword here is "wise." Processing the nuances of this relationship is key to moving forward. God knows you'd hate to repeat the experience, but one must slow down and take objective inventory.

I'll end this chapter with this anecdote. I was on a Southwest Airlines flight recently, and I'm an A-list member, so don't judge me. The flight attendant was walking us through the emergency protocols: Put your tray tables up, buckle up, and keep your 2-inch recline up; otherwise, you're in danger. Listen, Linda, we're all grown adults being instructed on how to buckle our seatbelts. I think we have a bigger problem if we haven't figured that out. But what was funny was I looked at her and decided this time I was going to listen. I don't know why, but I'm going to. And I thought to myself, *It's ironic; she's walking us through how to exit an airplane when things go south.* They really try to hone in on these details, warning us of what to do in case of an emergency. And yet, God forbid the plane ever crashes, the only thing people can think of is, *Get me out of this plane, and I'll be fine.*

The same goes for relationships. You think as long as you're out of this relationship, everything will be fine. But the funny thing is, you're on the other side waiting for yourself, so don't be so sure. **Repeating the pain is inevitable unless you get intentional**. This experience can and will happen again unless you get clear and make the unconscious, which dictates 90% of your choices, conscious.

> "You think as long as you're out of this relationship, everything will be fine. But the funny thing is, you're on the other side waiting for yourself, so don't be so sure."

There is a time and season for everything in life: a time to heal, a time to grieve, a time to mourn, and a time to laugh. For your sake, it's good to recognize the season you are in and honor it. **Remember, healing isn't linear—it's intentional.**

Reflection Questions:

1. What is your pattern that you somehow keep creating or attracting?

_____

_____

_____

_____

_____

_____

2. What's your process been in the past when a relationship ends?

　

3. What's the narrative you play like a podcast in your brain around this connection?

4. With curiosity and not judgment, what led you to the relationship originally?

5. What truly kept you in the relationship?

6. What did you tell yourself about them and about yourself?

___

7. What beliefs were revealed by this connection that were online before the connection?

___

8. Are you actually ready to rewire your brain to stop creating this painful experience?

   _____

   _____

   _____

   _____

   _____

   _____

9. What proactive steps can you put in place that will help the next time this comes up?

   _____

   _____

   _____

   _____

   _____

   _____

10. How do you grieve, if at all?

_____

_____

_____

_____

_____

_____

11. Are you willing to perceive a healthier approach to grieving?

_____

_____

_____

_____

_____

_____

12. What are the red flags I'm scared to acknowledge about myself or my partner?

___

13. What behavior in me has developed negatively or positively from this relationship?

___

14. How has this been like other relationships in the past?

15. What pain am I ignoring in myself, and what coping mechanisms have I created?

16. How do I make our relationship hard?

_____

_____

_____

_____

_____

_____

17. Am I willing to stay and become the best me, even if this person never changes?

_____

_____

_____

_____

_____

_____

18. What are the red flags I'm scared to acknowledge about myself or my partner?

_____

_____

_____

_____

_____

_____

19. What behavior in me has developed negatively or positively from this relationship?

_____

_____

_____

_____

_____

_____

20. How has this been like other relationships in the past?

_____

_____

_____

_____

_____

_____

21. What pain am I ignoring in myself, and what coping mechanisms have I created?

_____

_____

_____

_____

_____

_____

22. What beliefs keep me in this current relationship?

___

23. What work am I honestly willing to put in so that we have a better connection?

___

24. Do I want to work to connect deeper with this vulnerable human, intimately and proactively being fully open?

___

25. Outside of sex and security, what do I value about this relationship?

___

26. What am I most afraid of when ending this relationship?

_____
_____
_____
_____
_____
_____

27. What am I afraid of by staying?

_____
_____
_____
_____
_____
_____

28. What measurable actions and timelines do I need to set in order to maintain this connection?

_____

_____

_____

_____

_____

_____

29. What does forgiveness look like in order to move forward in life?

_____

_____

_____

_____

_____

_____

CHAPTER EIGHT
Wisdom From Painful Endings

No judgments here, but I imagine that as the tattoo "NO RAGRATS" is being inked across someone's chest, there will likely be second thoughts one day. It's indicative that a simple moment, a simple choice, can stay with you for quite a long time. Shame has no place in you if you want to create a life worth living. However, it is healthy to look back and reflect on what you might have done differently.

Imagine your friends are returning from participating in an active treasure hunt for something you've only heard of. As they're coming back, you're getting ready to leave and head to the place they've been. You notice two of them walking towards you, both bloodied and bandaged up. As they speak, you begin to listen, and everything else goes quiet. The exchange could save your life and hopefully help you find this treasure. All of this is based on your ability to listen and apply the wisdom they impart. So, you focus on every detail as if your life depends on it because, to some extent, it does.

I wonder if we'd be willing to treat relationships coming to an end in the same manner. I wonder if we'd be willing to be intentional about how much wisdom we could glean from other people's pain and their perspectives. Here's some potentially useful feedback from a few divorcees who may not have died on the side of a treacherous mountain trek, but they've definitely shared some insights during and after the ending of their relationships.

> *"I wonder if we'd be willing to be intentional about how much wisdom we could glean from other people's pain and their perspectives."*

Here are ten items that would have saved me from heartache shared by a 60-year-old divorcee:

1. I blamed my kid's father for most things; vengeance and manipulation drove me.

2. Controlling access to the kids wasn't my right, but somehow I got away with it. The children's welfare should have come before my agenda.

3. I wish I would have honored the other parent even if injustice had taken place. My narrative or pain wasn't their responsibility.

4. Don't involve your children in your conflict. Never degrade the other parent in front of or with your child.

5. Your emotions may be valid, but kids aren't built to carry your feelings. They'll resent you later if you do. Mine sure did.

6. Never get a divorce from another person without healing. Going broken into a new relationship isn't going to last. I should've healed, regardless of who I was with.

7. Make the decision to release and forgive them for the pain they may indirectly or directly cause you to experience.

8. Attachments to bitterness are stronger than love. It'll poison you and everyone around you, like drinking poison and wishing pain on others.

9. Give your heart time to breathe, rest, and heal. Skip dating for intentional season. Care for yourself. Spend time alone. You didn't end up here overnight.

10. The more you heal, the better equipped you'll be to help your children. Be deliberate in being present with them. Healing will take time for both them and you. Reestablishing a new family unit can take several years. Allow the children to express themselves without fear of repercussions. Don't control their narrative, but remind them it's not their fault.

As you read these stories, picture in your mind some of those regrets and ask yourself, *Could these apply to my life? Am I aware of this?*

"Avoidable mistakes I made" by a 37-year-old divorcee:

1. I didn't make a plan before I left. I waited too long and then left in a panic. I heeded the wrong legal advice. Ps, you can fire an attorney at any moment of engagement.

2. Keeping finances in check and getting clear on my money should have been a priority.

3. I wish I had unpacked my bags before going on another trip, relationally speaking.

4. Kill the social media feed. There's zero justification for it and no benefits.

5. I should have been more hyper-focused on healing and growth. I delayed the inevitable, the repetition of my pain, and it took several relationships to be revealed.

6. I wish I realized that my kids just needed me to be fully present and emotionally available, not have all the answers.

7. I listened to advice from people who hadn't been where I was or where I was going. I wasted so much time and energy defending my choice to friends and family. I wish I would have created more distance and boundaries with people who didn't support me.

8. It would have saved me an enormous amount of pain if I truly figured out my role and contribution to the relationship I left in the first place.

9. Grief is the most inconvenient gift you could ever give yourself. It might take longer or shorter than you expect, but don't hold it to a timeline.

10. Turning to emotional antibiotics like alcohol, drugs, and sex momentarily eased the aching; eventually, it made it worse.

11. Don't waste your time worrying about false narratives, lies, or gossip. They'll find another thing to talk about eventually.

12. Never ever talk about your ex to anyone. Say nothing in any direction.

13. The truth eventually gets revealed about people; let that happen on its own.

You see, **there is no laser surgery for bad decisions, but there is grace**. That grace comes online when you **own your contribution to the cycle and pivot**. You can go out and get the revenge body of a lifetime or become super independent, but if we're honest, it's mostly out of ego and insecurity. If you're pursuing health, do it because you actually care about yourself.

The relationship you're leaving has marked you, both by being in it and leaving it. It's up to you whether it marks you for better or worse. The beauty lies in exchanging pain for healing, growth, and forgiveness. Forgive them and forgive yourself. Shame is paralyzing and can lead to making bad decisions in the future without realizing it. People often say, "Oh, I'll never get married again. All men are trash, or they're all players or narcissists."

A side note: only 1% of the population are actually narcissists, so skip the pop psychology of branding your exes. Just take ownership of your actions and your roles, whatever they were in the connection. You'd be surprised at the feedback you'd receive if you asked people for an honest reflection on how you could have shown up better. I'm not telling you to chase down your abusive ex for feedback, but seeking input from people you still respect isn't a bad idea. It's not for the faint of heart, but there can be some brutally honest nuggets if you look for truth in what they're saying. You'll be surprised at the feedback some people give you, especially the quiet ones.

> *"You'd be surprised at the feedback you'd receive if you asked people for an honest reflection on how you could have shown up better."*

I literally say to myself, *How can I prove what they're saying is true? Where's the gold in what they're saying?* It might not be the absolute truth, but there is gold in there, and **I'm going to take it and grow, even at the cost of my ego.**

Every week, I watch my daughter come back from pottery classes with something new she has created. Sometimes, in disappointment, she would tell me, "This piece isn't for anything but learning; I have no practical use for it. I want to toss it in the trash, but I'll remember next time where I went wrong. My teacher said that it's okay to create something I don't want, just for the sake of creating." (Cue slow clapping, proud father moment.)

It's mesmerizing and soothing to watch a potter create a piece from raw clay, water, and intention. Life shapes and molds us, much like how people and painful events shape us. The pain of life acts as a fire, hardening the molding of one's heart. But here's the beauty: you can add water and get back on the potter's wheel, only to be made into something beautiful. This isn't a one-time defeat or failure. Fail forward.

I'm sure that some of you absolutely love, admire, and respect your parents. Maybe some of you reading this are absolutely committed to never being anything like your parents. It's funny; when you want to ensure that you're never like them, there are traits you actually carry that are just like them, possibly toxic, and you don't even know it. There's gold in your backyard. If you're willing to dig it up and cash it in, **pain can be as valuable as gold.** Your own relationships showcase your perceived value. See, we train people not only how to treat us, but we also train ourselves how to respond. When we're young, we act out of survival and the need for acceptance. And those things shape our personal reality, which we call our personality.

This chapter, aimed at helping you avoid massive regrets, is really just encouraging you to commit to your inner growth, regardless of who's on the other side of the partnership with you or if you're single.

If you're reading this, it means, to some extent, you want more for yourself. I'm telling you, the real answer is not whether or not you stay in a relationship. It's how committed you are to your growth and authentic wholeness because **you're going to have to live with yourself for the rest of your life.** If you stay, you have to face your inner world and no longer ignore the alarms going off. I think you get the picture I'm painting.

Start by learning how to love yourself well, which begins with embracing uncomfortable truths. This is a precise indicator of cognitive dissonance—whether one is ready to engage with differing viewpoints. While it may be challenging, being open to new information and considering its application is crucial. Note that this process requires curiosity rather than self-hatred, judgment, or shame. A client once contacted me, struggling with a breakthrough, unable to achieve the desired outcome. It became evident that he was treating himself harshly, essentially holding himself emotionally captive with self-judgment for not attaining his expected goals. Surprisingly, we all carry a burden of self-judgment or preconceived notions about ourselves, acting as beacons that signal the world to reinforce these negative beliefs. Essentially, it's as if we're saying, "This is what I believe about myself, so please continue to validate my self-hatred."

There's a high likelihood that your partnership was formed based on who you thought you were in the past. You constructed an identity tower on beliefs that no longer benefit you, and that realization is frightening. With every tremor, this collapsing house of cards reveals more about your true self. Who are you? What do you believe in? How did you end up here? It's time to meticulously remove every part of yourself that no longer serves you, and that, my friend, takes time. Your identity requires a new foundation. To achieve this, everything built on this false sense of self must fall. You're welcome because although it may feel like the painful yet relieving sensation of waxing nose hairs—tears might flow—you'll ultimately breathe more easily, I assure you. Like the controlled demolition of a building, it can be messy, but with intentionality, collateral damage can be minimized. You can safely bring down a large building in the heart of downtown when done correctly. Similarly, placing your identity and value in something that no longer suits you won't destroy you as a person. Rebuilding your value and identity on new grounds might leave you feeling raw and vulnerable for a while.

> *"It's time to meticulously remove every part of yourself that no longer serves you, and that, my friend, takes time. Your identity requires a new foundation. To achieve this, everything built on this false sense of self must fall."*

Sometimes, couples outgrow each other, and it becomes a learning experience about ourselves as individuals. For your sake and the sake of possible future partners, don't waste it. I advise both men and women—don't squander this pain. Extract as much value from it as possible. It can teach you a great deal if you know how to "squeeze the lemon," so to speak. You are not defined by your pain. You may have experienced it, but your identity doesn't reside in it. **Rather, pain reflects a part of your identity that needs adjustment. Clean those lenses and heal the wounds that have shaped you.** Strive to become the best version of yourself. Hold yourself to a higher standard.

Reflection Questions:

1. What are my obvious regrets in past relationships?

_____

_____

_____

_____

_____

_____

_____

2. What belief is my pain trying to reveal that I believe and don't realize it?

___

3. After I realized I made a mistake, how long did it take to pivot or change directions?

___

4. **Am I willing to proactively acknowledge pain long before regret?**

5. **What does it look like to build self-trust?**

6. Does life feel intentional or a passive roller coaster? What's this revealing about me?

___

7. How many times in the last week did you look in the mirror before leaving the house or walking into an appointment? Am I examining my thoughts as vigorously as my image?

___

As you contemplate how you present yourself to the world, consider why we do not look inward with the same vigor and intentionality to examine our hearts and emotional health. **True self-awareness is an art and a massive pursuit worthy of your efforts.** If you're not growing in some capacity, you're digressing.

CHAPTER NINE

Prove This Wrong

It's time to acquire the house of your dreams. The builder sits across from you, offering two houses for sale. The first house is located on a brand new road at 101 West Good Intentions Avenue. It boasts a beautiful, brand-new front door, and inside, you'll find oak cabinets with carpet from the 80s. It's definitely not been worked on much, but there's a familiarity to it. Although the foundation has some cracks and it leaks a bit when it rains, the fresh coat of paint looks pretty. Just a block away, a custom-remodeled home awaits at 200 Dream Lane. Its windows, roof, HVAC, and appliances are state-of-the-art, requiring no future replacements. However, this home is more expensive than the first, and you must wait six months for completion before moving in. Which home would you choose? If it's cheap enough, most would choose the old home in the name of cost. In reality, it's the potential we buy into, like most people. Relationships are based upon two people's efforts, sure, but "don't go chasing waterfalls" doesn't begin to describe how low our standards get just because something is available and requires little investment, emotionally speaking.

Many of us hastily journey down the path to relational turmoil, paved with good intentions. Ironically, if we evaluated our decision-making process with utmost intentionality, our relationships would resemble a well-designed home. It's often easier to be paranoid and opt to "stay single" due to fear of getting hurt or facing disappointment again.

I've distilled this guide into four main lenses, four concepts, or four pillars—akin to a four-legged table—to apply to any relationship or connection in your life. Have you ever tried sitting on a two-legged stool? It would be unstable, prone to slight movements, and ill-suited to support anything of value.

We often build romantic connections or friendships without an intentionally built foundation. These four key lenses for evaluating relationships will determine whether a connection has the potential to last and flourish.

1. **Get clear on your values and live in them without apology**. Learn how to create affiliation minus emotional intimacy whenever there aren't shared values, as unshared values will become a source of conflict.

2. **Become deadly at managing and setting clear expectations**. Bids reveal our needs, and the responses from our partners are crucial on both sides. Mismanaged expectations create resentment 100% of the time towards ourselves or our partner. Yes, you should definitely have expectations, and they should be clearly established and frequently revisited between the two of you.

3. **Stay vigilant in how you show up and handle conflict when it arises**. Conflict management is an invaluable skill. Calling time out, pausing, or acknowledging the unspoken tension is a gift to

everyone involved. Getting clear on how to manage disconnection and coming back together is your gift to the relationship.

4. **Chemistry is a must,** especially when it's not based on toxic, unsafe behavior. Entire books are written on keeping the fire stoked with seduction and healthy passion inside of a relationship. Being playful, seductive, and pursuing your partner are essential ingredients for the relationship's survival. If these elements are missing, you're heading towards a sex desert.

When you intentionally cultivate all four of these ideas in a relationship, it's inevitable that the relationship will flourish as a legendary unicorn flying over rainbows. You're welcome for the visual.

I'm waiting for someone to fully apply these principles, yet there's still an inexplicable breakdown in their friendship or connections. Nine times out of ten, we can usually identify one or more of these principles as the culprit when a relationship ends. Once these four are understood and applied, everything changes—every single connection in your life. The most common issues we see in relationships are related to expectations and values. There's a cyclical relationship among all *four pillars*. **Conflict Management** leads to **Chemistry**, which then delves into **Expectations** and **Values**, bringing us right back to conflict. If we tip one of these pillars over, it's going to affect or be supported by the others.

> *"Once these four are understood and applied, everything changes—every single connection in your life. The most common issues we see in relationships are related to expectations and values."*

Have you ever wished you could guide someone you know towards addressing the elephant in the room that's holding them back? You cannot desire growth for others more than they want it for themselves. Likely, their journey will look different from what you think it should look like in every way. The best gift you can give those around you is to **do your own work,** process your pain, own your wounds, programs, and triggers that drive your behavior. Face your ego. Dethrone the false self that has kept you safe for so long. Heal the hidden parts of you.

Remember, it's like returning a well-served ball for you pickleball enthusiasts. Your response can significantly change because it comes from a changed space: you. This is quite empowering when you think about it.

I used to be skeptical of online courses because I always felt like I overpaid in the end. However, I decided to create an intensive deep dive into what it looks like to apply these principles in one's life. What is shared in this group setting stays there. It's an opportunity to see others and be seen to the extent of vulnerability you choose. No one's work is solely their own. As you process your issues, others are doing the exact same work, which will amplify the emotional return on investment throughout the experience.

If you're married, this will expose your marriage's weak points and help you grow. If you're going through a divorce or are about to, the course is perfect for you to process this with someone who has the scars and strength to hold space alongside you. If you want to potentially marry someone who is near and dear to your heart, this should be the standard that helps determine that leap.

This isn't for everyone or the faint of heart. If you are easily offended or haven't begun this type of work, I encourage you to read this twice and truly delve into the methods I mentioned. There is no greater gift to the world than the act of authentic self-love first. They tell you to put on your oxygen mask first on an airplane for a reason. **I have no greater honor and respect for people than when they pursue ownership, growth, and healing.** I commend you because if it were easy, everyone would do this work.

HERE'S A "TO GO" GIFT

I'm going to give you a **Checklist for Your Relationship.** If you don't score an 8/10 in all four categories, it should become an intentional focus of the relationship. Consider it the new "check engine" light of your relationship, okay? These four markers are designed to create the best possible chance for a safe, fulfilling, and thriving relationship. I have observed a relationship "survive" on merely two out of the four, but that's the limit. It usually reflects an unspoken survival mode in most cases.

Getting to know yourself is quite an intentional pursuit, similar to peeling back the layers of an onion (it's okay if there are tears). There are likely unhealed wounds that have yet to be processed. Well, you need to address these, as they're reflected in your relationships of all kinds. This book is not the ultimate solution for life but a contender for what I consider the best relationship advice out there. It's what rudiments are to a drummer, drills are to an athlete, and **foundations are to anything worth building.**

I've created a course where I share the deeper parts of each chapter. It breaks down the why and the return on investment of deploying these lenses to your relational outlook. It comes with a one-on-one coaching session, where I hold space with you through some straightforward, possibly intensive conversations. We're putting together couples retreats as I type this, which will be monumental. I had judgments toward those who created courses, but with all my heart, I wish someone had shared this stuff with me. It would've saved me tens of thousands of dollars and years of gut-wrenching therapy. Don't get me wrong, healing is worth it, no question about it. **There are two teachers in life: pain and wisdom from others. Honor and heal the pain you've already experienced. Act upon the wisdom imparted from others without the cost of pain. Leverage my pain.**

Simplified Relational Checklist:

Your current relationship status doesn't dictate your posture towards this content. If you're divorced or going through a breakup, your responsibility is to process everything and transform it into fertilizer from the relationship. What worked, what didn't, and why? Step out of your typical interpretation of the relationship and become objective. One way I've found to achieve this is through feedback from an outside perspective, from someone who you consider emotionally safe.

1. **List out some objective ways in which you showed up or tolerated that didn't work in benefit of the connection.**

   _____

   _____

   _____

   _____

2. If you are married and wish to increase sustainability, it's time to clarify each other's values. Are you both willing to work on cultivating healthier chemistry, better conflict management, and managing expectations? Are you willing to grow in these areas, even if you're focused on solo growth?

_____

_____

_____

_____

3. How would you rate YOURSELF and your partner during the previous or current relationship? Where are you lacking in these four areas as an individual and as a couple?

_____

_____

_____

_____

4. How do you rate you and your partners' relational pillars?

_____

_____

_____

_____

_____

a) Do you have shared values and/or are willing to honor one another's values?
b) Giving and responding to Bids, Booty Calls, and Boundaries: 1 - 10 _____.
c) Conflict Management willingness, skills, and ability: 1 - 10 _____.
d) Healthy intentionally cultivated Chemistry: 1 - 10 _____.

When we avoid hard conversations with ourselves or someone else, we trade short-term discomfort for long-term dysfunction.

Remember this: if you do not face your pain, you will create a much greater one for yourself.

THANK YOU FOR READING MY BOOK!

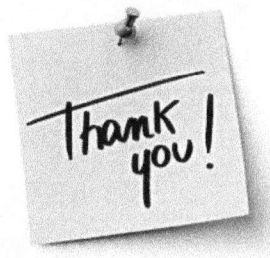

Thank you for reading my book! Here is a free bonus.

Change your life now!

I appreciate your interest in my book and value your feedback as it helps me improve future versions of this book. I would appreciate it if you could leave your invaluable review on Amazon.com with your feedback. Thank you!